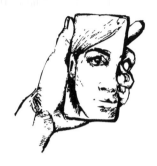

NARCISSISM AND ITS DISCONTENTS

Diagnostic Dilemmas and Treatment Strategies With Narcissistic Patients

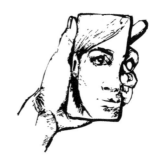

NARCISSISM AND ITS DISCONTENTS

Diagnostic Dilemmas and Treatment Strategies With Narcissistic Patients

Glen O. Gabbard, M.D.
Holly Crisp, M.D.

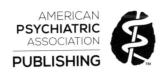

AMERICAN
PSYCHIATRIC
ASSOCIATION
PUBLISHING

If you wish to buy 50 or more copies of the same title, please go to www.appi.org/specialdiscounts for more information.

Copyright © 2018 American Psychiatric Association Publishing

ALL RIGHTS RESERVED

First Edition

Manufactured in the United States of America on acid-free paper
25 24 23   5 4 3

American Psychiatric Association Publishing
800 Maine Ave. SW, Suite 900
Washington, DC 20024-2812
www.appi.org

Library of Congress Cataloging-in-Publication Data
Names: Gabbard, Glen O., author. | Crisp, Holly, author. | American
  Psychiatric Association Publishing, publisher.
Title: Narcissism and its discontents : diagnostic dilemmas and treatment
  strategies with narcissistic patients / Glen O. Gabbard, Holly Crisp.
Description: First edition. | Washington, D.C. : American Psychiatric
  Association Publishing, [2018] | Includes bibliographical references and
  index.
Identifiers: LCCN 2018001808 (print) | LCCN 2018002297 (ebook) |
  ISBN 9781615371938 (eb) | ISBN 9781615371273 (pb : alk. paper)
Subjects: | MESH: Narcissism | Personality Disorders—therapy | Personality
  Disorders—diagnosis | Treatment Outcome | Physician-Patient Relations
Classification: LCC RC553.N36 (ebook) | LCC RC553.N36 (print) | NLM WM
  460.5.E3 | DDC 616.85/854—dc23
LC record available at https://lccn.loc.gov/2018001808

British Library Cataloguing in Publication Data
A CIP record is available from the British Library.

Contents

About the Authors vii

Disclosure of Interests ix

Preface xi

Part I
Diagnostic Dilemmas

1 Narcissism and Its Discontents 3

2 The Cultural Context of Narcissism 19

3 Modes of Relatedness 33

Part II
Treatment Strategies

4 Beginning the Treatment 57

5 Transference and Countertransference 77

6 Tailoring the Treatment to the Patient 97

7 Treatment Strategies 117

8 Termination 139

Index. 153

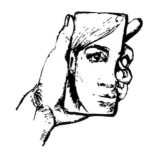

About the Authors

Glen O. Gabbard, M.D., is Clinical Professor of Psychiatry at Baylor College of Medicine in Houston, Texas. He is also Training and Supervising Analyst at the Center for Psychoanalytic Studies in Houston. He is in the full-time private practice of psychiatry, psychoanalysis, and psychotherapy.

Holly Crisp, M.D., is Clinical Associate Professor at Baylor College of Medicine in Houston, Texas. She is on the faculty at the Center for Psychoanalytic Studies in Houston. She is in the full-time private practice of psychiatry, psychoanalysis, and psychotherapy.

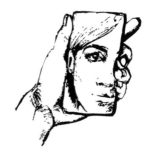

Disclosure of Interests

The authors have indicated that they have no financial interests or other affiliations that represent or could appear to represent a competing interest with their contributions to this book.

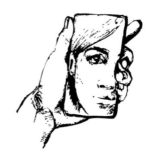

Preface

While we were preparing this book, which is written for clinicians who face the challenges of narcissistically organized patients, we became aware that a certain fascination with narcissists had emerged within the recent discourse on politics and celebrity. The popular culture today is replete with visions of narcissism—for better or worse. In many ways, narcissistic personality disorder has been garnering the interest that once surrounded borderline personality disorder. Which public figures are truly narcissistic? Can mental health professionals dare to diagnose them? Is narcissism necessary for success? Have social media and smartphones generated a culture of self-absorbed navel-gazers who are incapable of connecting to others?

We do not have all the answers to these questions. Our focus is clearly on the clinical picture of patients struggling with narcissistic issues and how mental health professionals might approach them. Hence, we devote only one chapter to the new culture of narcissism. Moreover, our book is not a comprehensive treatment guide but rather an exploration of common dilemmas that occur in clinical work with narcissistically organized individuals and a host of strategies to deal with those dilemmas in the treatment setting.

In our psychiatric practices, we have seen a great many patients with narcissistic issues over the years. As psychoanalysts, our approach to treatment, whatever form it may take, is based on the perspective of contemporary psychoanalytic thinking, which starts with what is particular, unique, and idiosyncratic about the individual. This book evolved from years of work with specific narcissistically organized individuals who did not fit neatly into one category or another. This work led to the growing realization that narcissism is actually pleomorphic, a multiheaded hydra with a multiplicity of forms.

Our work is also informed by research data on narcissism, which we attempt to integrate with our clinical understanding. We examine empirical research data from attachment theory, large surveys of populations, and psychotherapy studies. Much of the literature on this subject features psychoanalysis proper as the treatment of choice, but the vast majority of patients do not have access to that treatment. Thus, although we discuss psychoanalysis as a treatment, we also address psychotherapeutic strategies that are less intensive than analysis but also useful. Finally, we outline general strategies for treating narcissistic patients, including the use of transference and countertransference, that are applicable to all treatment settings, whether pharmacotherapy, partial hospital, or inpatient.

We recognize that narcissistic personality disorder is not well understood. It is a moving target that can vary from day to day in the same person. There is also a spectrum from healthy to pathological narcissism. Different approaches may be necessary to address the various locations on the continuum. Some forms of narcissism are regarded as developmentally "normal" at a particular age while appearing pathological at another. Differentiating healthy from pathological narcissism is a difficult process. Also, applying the diagnosis of narcissistic personality disorder can be complicated. Some narcissistically organized individuals may appear monotonously the same and oblivious to the therapist sitting in the room with them, whereas others may carefully observe the therapist with laser beam scrutiny. We suggest that narcissism is highly reactive to specific contexts and in some cases may vary considerably from one appointment to the next. As psychoanalytic clinicians, we think the best approach to the diagnosis and treatment of narcissistically organized patients is to look for what is idiosyncratic and unique about the person with the condition rather than applying a "one-size-fits-all" approach.

A thoughtful, individualized approach is necessary in order to take into account the specific features of the person sitting in the patient's chair. Manualized treatments are necessary for rigorous research but may stifle the therapist's creativity in clinical practice. We strongly believe that the therapist or analyst conducting the treatment needs to be flexible. Tailoring the therapy to the patient may require a series of trial-and-error modifications of one's technique. There is also a process within the clinician of finding one's own voice suited to the person of the patient but also reflective of who the person of the therapist is (Gabbard and Ogden 2009). Experienced psychoanalysts and psychoanalytic therapists discover at some point that they are not quite the same as they proceed from one patient to another in the course of a work day. We all re-create ourselves to some extent from one hour to the next. With narcissistic patients in particular, clinicians must retain flexibility. Moreover, the gender of the patient and the therapist may create unique challenges that deserve more attention in the literature on treatment. Hence, the contributions of a male and a female coauthor are useful in a text such as this one.

In this volume, we hope to engage the reader in an intersubjective process of adjusting the treatment to the patient rather than forcing the patient into a slot that may be problematic for the patient's subjectivity. Narcissistic patients spend their lives trying to find someone who can see them, hear them, and "get" them. We hope to promote this imperfect, but always worthwhile, search for a useful "fit" between what the patient may need and what the therapist may offer.

We wish to thank Jill Craig for her highly skilled typing, editing, and fact checking. We also want to thank Dr. Laura Roberts, Editor-in-Chief, and John McDuffie, Interim Publisher, at American Psychiatric Association Publishing for their support and wise counsel. We also thank our many teachers and mentors who taught us how to approach patients as complex human beings who yearn to be understood rather than diagnostic entities who must be classified. And finally, we owe a debt of gratitude to our patients who have taught us so much about narcissism and its origins.

Glen O. Gabbard, M.D.
Holly Crisp, M.D.

Houston, Texas, 2018

REFERENCE

Gabbard GO, Ogden TH: On becoming a psychoanalyst. Int J Psychoanal 90(2):311–327, 2009 19382962

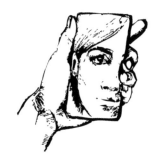

Part I

Diagnostic Dilemmas

1

Narcissism and Its Discontents

Today, the discontents of narcissism are all around us. First and foremost, many patients with narcissistic disturbances are unhappy. They often live lives of noisy desperation. They cannot seem to find what they are seeking. In fact, they are not even certain about what it is they hope to find. The notion of self-love is often used to characterize the essence of narcissism, but it applies to only a subgroup of individuals with pathological narcissism. More often, narcissists are extraordinarily insecure about their capacity to love and be loved and are frantic in their search for others who will admire them, be impressed by them, empathize with their needs, validate their specialness, and/or serve as an idealized object who will never shame them or humiliate them. However, they tend to go through life disappointed because what they seek is a tall order—one that usually cannot be fulfilled in a world of imperfect, ambivalent relationships.

The level of suffering in persons with narcissistic disturbances is highly variable. Some have constructed defensive facades such that they avoid—at least partially—the distress over their emptiness or their incapacity to obtain the response they wish from others. Others go through life with an open wound, feeling like they are being attacked from every direction, with no respite from the pain. Many are on a continuum between the two extremes, with variations that depend on current stressors and specific contexts in their lives. In any case, it would be safe to assume that the majority are unhappy, if not despairing.

Mental health professionals engaged in clinical work find the term *narcissism* vexing because they cannot be certain of what is meant when a colleague speaks of narcissism. Does pathological narcissism denote too much self-love? Profound insecurity? Low self-esteem? Too much self-esteem? Selfishness? Aloofness? A conviction that one is smarter, better looking, more fashionable, or better connected than others? An inability to tune in to what others are feeling or thinking? Used as an adjective, *narcissistic* may refer to someone who is thoroughly unpleasant and obnoxious or someone whose success and confidence are envied.

Almost everyone recognizes the existence of such a thing as healthy self-interest, that is, a kind of narcissism that involves self-care and pride in a job well done. Whether a self-serving behavior is pathological or not may also depend on the phase of one's life cycle. An adolescent girl who spends hours obsessing about how she wishes to appear in the photo she is about to upload to social media may well be seen as "normal" for her stage in life. To complicate matters further, one person labeled "narcissistic" may respond to a slight by having an emotional meltdown, whereas another with the same label may appear to be impervious to any insult because of his seeming self-confidence. This widespread confusion about the nature of narcissism—both healthy and pathological—clearly reflects the fact that there are many faces of narcissism (Burgo 2015; Caligor et al. 2015; Campbell and Miller 2011; Gabbard and Crisp-Han 2016).

The discontent of clinicians is also linked to the frustration they experience with their attempts to treat narcissistic patients, who may insist on dictating the conditions of treatment, ignore the comments of their therapists, and "correct" their therapists by indicating to them where they have gone wrong and pointing out what they should say and when they should say it. Moreover, these patients are often frustrating because they disappear from treatment abruptly without explanation. On the other end of the continuum, when they stick with therapy, the treatment may be protracted with very little sign of change. Indeed, these patients may seem impervious to the observations of the clinician treating them and yet stay in treatment without making substantial improvements. These treatments may be among the longest and most arduous and may seem interminable.

Researchers in the mental health field can also be included among the discontents. Narcissistic personality disorder (NPD) as a clinical entity has been challenging to study. Because of the pleomorphic nature of NPD, defining the entity for meaningful research has tried the minds of a host of skilled researchers. When the American Psychiatric Association Personality Disorders Work Group assembled to develop criteria for DSM-5 (American Psychiatric Association 2013), this body suggested that NPD should be deleted from DSM-5 because of its low prevalence and the paucity of systematic research on NPD compared with many of the other personality disorders (Skodol et al. 2011). Intense debate continued about which entities should or should not be included in the DSM-5 personality disorders, fueled by a recommendation on the part of the Personality Disorders Work Group to revamp the system for specific diagnostic criteria. At the same time, scores of clinicians and researchers were outraged at the notion of dropping NPD from the DSM-5 group of personality disorders because of its high prevalence in clinical practice. Despite the lack of clarity and rigorous research, NPD as a diagnosis was ultimately included among the DSM-5 personality disorders, much to the relief of many clinicians.

Families of young adults who have the NPD diagnosis are a third category of discontents. It has become a common practice in contemporary mental health care for clinicians to sit down with the patient and family and explain the basis for the diagnosis as part of a psychoeducational intervention designed to provide useful information. In many cases, such as borderline personality disorder, this approach has led to a more sophisticated and effective approach to treatment where families and patients can ally themselves in a systematic effort to improve the symptoms and the quality of life of the patient (Gunderson and Hoffman 2005). However, when it comes to the diagnosis of NPD, neither patients nor families want to hear those three words as the diagnostic conclusion of the evaluating professional. Because the term *narcissistic* has such a pejorative connotation in its use throughout society, it is rarely received by a patient or a family as a useful piece of information that can direct treatment. Sharing that information often results in explosive anger, hurt feelings, denial, and blaming. The diagnosis may connote to the patient that he or she is a dreadful person and cause a descent into profound shame and humiliation.

Lovers and spouses are yet another group of disgruntled individuals who feel they have been profoundly mistreated by narcissistic individuals. Dombek (2016) noted that the widespread shift of contemporary discourse to cyberspace has provided a place for victims of narcissists to share their experience and receive support from others. Web sites where people can go for support include www.narcissismsurvivor.com, www.narcissismuncovered.com, www.thenarcissisticlife.com, and www.narcissismfree.com. Many of the depictions featured at these Web sites provide horrific portraits of the selfishness of people with narcissistic features and heartbreaking accounts of those who have been mistreated by them. They also serve as support groups for those who feel they have been taken advantage of by severely self-centered spouses or lovers. Books written for lay readers have also appeared that provide guidance to those who feel they need help in extricating themselves from narcissistic relationships (Beharry 2013; Burgo 2015). Hence, there appears to be a relatively large contingent of discontents who are up in arms about their victimization at the hands of narcissistic victimizers.

This opening overview of the discontents omits a rarely discussed aspect inherent in the treatment of narcissistic patients: the distinct pleasure that clinicians may feel with some narcissistically organized patients who convey a desperate wish to be loved and known that evokes empathy, admiration, and human connection. With such patients, a fundamental credo of clinicians, which is to relieve the patient's suffering, comes to the fore.

THE MYTH OF NARCISSUS

Psychoanalysts have been fond of appropriating ancient texts from Greek and Roman authors in their exposition of syndromes they see in clinical practice. Sophocles provided the tragedy of Oedipus. Ovid wrote of Narcissus. In the Narcissus myth, which has a number of variations, a boy looks into a pool of water and falls in love with his own reflection. This oversimplified version, however, is probably not what Ovid intended. In fact, Narcissus thinks he sees another boy, not himself. Narcissus is overwhelmed with his experience of finding a perfect partner with whom an ideal love can exist. He experiences an ideal harmony in which two perfectly suited and perfectly identical people are united in bliss.

In Dombek's (2016) analysis of the myth, she noted that the story of Narcissus is actually a cautionary tale about the imperfect capacity to "know oneself." She stressed that we can fall into illusions when we find ourselves everywhere. From her perspective, the narrative of the myth is often incorrectly regarded as a portrayal of evil or pathology, but it is fundamentally a case of mistaken identities, that is, the illusions that we pass through on the way to love. Narcissists cannot see that they are looking at their own face when they think they are looking at someone else. The myth, then, is more about misrecognition than self-love. Ovid's story is about someone who looks at another person and sees an idealized version of himself and then falls in love with a reflection rather than a person.

THE MULTIHEADED HYDRA OF NARCISSISM

The problem of coming to a clear consensus on the nature of NPD or pathological narcissism arises out of its varied presentations and the diversity of the individuals who may receive the diagnosis. The DSM-5 criteria set for NPD is misleading in this regard (Box 1–1).

Box 1–1. DSM-5 Diagnostic Criteria for Narcissistic Personality Disorder   **301.81** (F60.81)

A pervasive pattern of grandiosity (in fantasy or behavior), need for admiration, and lack of empathy, beginning by early adulthood and present in a variety of contexts, as indicated by five (or more) of the following:

1. Has a grandiose sense of self-importance (e.g., exaggerates achievements and talents, expects to be recognized as superior without commensurate achievements).
2. Is preoccupied with fantasies of unlimited success, power, brilliance, beauty, or ideal love.
3. Believes that he or she is "special" and unique and can only be understood by, or should associate with, other special or high-status people (or institutions).
4. Requires excessive admiration.
5. Has a sense of entitlement (i.e., unreasonable expectations of especially favorable treatment or automatic compliance with his or her expectations).
6. Is interpersonally exploitative (i.e., takes advantage of others to achieve his or her own ends).
7. Lacks empathy: is unwilling to recognize or identify with the feelings and needs of others.
8. Is often envious of others or believes that others are envious of him or her.
9. Shows arrogant, haughty behaviors or attitudes.

Source. Reprinted from American Psychiatric Association: *Diagnostic and Statistical Manual of Mental Disorders*, 5th Edition, Arlington, VA, American Psychiatric Association, 2013. Copyright © 2013 American Psychiatric Association. Used with permission.

These criteria are perhaps the ones most widely recognized by individuals inside and outside the mental health field—the bragging, self-important boor who wants everyone to admire him and "feed his ego." He or she may appear oblivious to the opinions of others and hide behind a veritable coat of armor that provides protection from feeling hurt or slighted (Gabbard 2014). The notion that five of the nine criteria will define NPD is oversimplified. The criteria may help in identifying one variant of pathological narcissism, but the multiheaded hydra of narcissism defies simple definitions that are based on the number of symptoms in a checklist.

A more nuanced subtyping has occurred in the past two decades that has allowed the field to endorse a grandiose or oblivious subtype on the one hand and a vulnerable or hypervigilant subtype on the other (Dickinson and Pincus 2003; Gabbard 1989, 1998; Pincus and Lukowitsky 2010; Wink 1991). In fact, as long ago as 1987, the British psychoanalyst Herbert Rosenfeld made a distinction between *thick-skinned* and *thin-skinned* narcissists. The vulnerable or hypervigilant individual is thin-skinned in that he or she is always perceiving slights or narcissistic injuries in the comments of others (Rosenfeld 1987). This subtype of narcissists may explode in emotional outbursts when feeling wounded. By contrast, the grandiose type is more oblivious to what is going on with others and sees those around him as potential audience members who may give him the admiration he needs.

This distinction between subtypes drawn from research and descriptive psychiatry is mirrored in the classic psychoanalytic writings of Otto Kernberg and Heinz Kohut. Kernberg's (1975) early clinical descriptions are similar to the grandiose, self-centered, and aggressive subtype. Kohut (1971, 1977) emphasized that narcissistic patients are developmentally arrested at a stage at which they require specific responses from persons in their environment in order to maintain a cohesive self. Empathic failures in the parents lead to fragmentations of the self. Hence, aggression in the patient would be regarded as secondary to narcissistic injuries from others. The self of a narcissistically organized person is seen as fragile but potentially "normal" if provided with empathy and compassion. Missing functions need to be internalized from others. Kernberg (1975, 1984, Kernberg 2014) emphasized that the self of a narcissistic individual is a highly pathological structure based on a conflict model, but Kohut's thinking is based on a deficit model in which the self is not a defensive structure.

Therapists conducting treatments with narcissistic patients have their own version of discontent when trying to "fit" their patients into concise diagnostic subtypes. These subtype distinctions risk an oversimplification of complex clinical presentations. Those patients who appear to be grandiose, self-confident, narcissistic individuals may fall apart in response to disappointments, rejections, or advancing age (Caligor et al. 2015; Gabbard 2014). Similarly, those who are hypervigilant may erupt into explosions of rage, contempt, and grandiosity if the narcissistic injury strikes a sensitive target within. Hence, these distinctions can depend on the moment in time when the narcissistic patient is seen. These subtypes also are problematic in that many of the studies leading to these conclusions were based heavily on self-report questionnaires. Research suggests that most individuals with personality disorders, and those with NPDs in particular, have little insight into how others experience them. Carlson and Oltmanns (2015) studied a large community sample of adults to determine which people might have personality disorder symptoms. Compared with the individuals in the study who had fewer personality disorder symptoms, those with more symptoms typical of personality disorder were less accurate in estimating the negativity of the impressions they made on their acquaintances. Hence, the authors concluded that this cohort with personality problems had difficulties with meta-perception.

To address this difficulty of overreliance on self-report questionnaires, Russ et al. (2008) used the Shedler-Westen Assessment Procedure-II (SWAP-II) to survey how clinicians made a diagnosis of NPD. Twelve hundred psychiatrists and clinical psychologists participated and used the SWAP-II to characterize patients who they felt were most characteristic of NPD. Hence, the prototypes gathered were based on clinical perspectives rather than self-report. From this exercise, a total of 255 patients met DSM-IV (American Psychiatric Association 1994) criteria for NPD. Q-factor analysis was used to identify three subtypes, which the authors labeled as grandiose/malignant, fragile, and high-functioning/exhibitionistic. They also found that core features of NPD include interpersonal vulnerability, difficulties regulating affect, competitiveness, and underlying emotional distress, all of which are absent from the DSM-5 criteria.

The *grandiose/malignant* type, or the oblivious narcissist, was characterized by exaggerated self-importance, lack of remorse, interpersonal manipulativeness, seething anger, pursuit of interpersonal power, and feelings of privilege. Persons in the *fragile* category, closely resembling the hypervigilant or vulnerable subtype, warded off painful feelings of inadequacy with grandiosity used defensively and had a powerful undercurrent of inadequate feelings, negative affect states, and loneliness. The clinicians whose reports were gathered also noted a considerable amount of shifting back and forth between grandiose feelings and inadequate feelings that reflected an alternation of contradictory self-representations triggered by varieties of threat. The third type, the *high-functioning* variant, had an exaggerated sense of self-importance, but these individuals were also outgoing, energetic, and articulate. They apparently had used their narcissism as strong motivation to succeed. They tended to be interpersonally adept and achievement oriented.

More recently, Ackerman et al. (2017) tried to clarify the definition of narcissism as used by both clinical psychologists and social/personality psychologists. A comprehensive list of attributes associated with narcissism was compiled, and experts from both disciplines rated the characteristics in terms of their centrality to narcissism. There was general agreement that grandiose features were most central. The key features rated by both groups of experts included a sense of entitlement, overly ambitious goals and ideals, grandiose fantasies, narcissistic rage, and hypervigilance. The fact that hypervigilance made the cut suggests that vulnerability to slights is recognized as a key factor in the diagnosis.

From a psychoanalytic perspective, a theme that runs across all subtypes of narcissistic patients is a concern about being seen by others and how they come across to those who see them. Steiner (2006) attributes this concern to an acute self-consciousness and a fear of being humiliated or shamed. Fragile or hypervigilant narcissists attempt to maintain self-esteem and avoid humiliating situations by tuning into others and figuring out how to behave. Oblivious or grandiose narcissists try to insulate themselves from narcissistic injury by screening out the responses of others (Gabbard 2014).

A common thread found in narcissistic disturbances is a sense of "lack." This can be viewed as lacking a sense of self that is durable and continuous through time, leading individuals to feel empty. Caligor et al. (2015) noted that an extremely fragile sense of self can be present, but it depends on the view of oneself as being exceptional in some way. By feeling grandiose or special, such individuals can have an illusion of some form of stable self-experience. Narcissistic colleagues or acquaintances are often referred to with comments such as "he is so full of himself!" The irony is that these individuals are often terribly empty (Dombek 2016).

FALSE DIALECTICS

A common dilemma faced by clinicians who are attempting to diagnose a narcissistic problem in a patient occurs when the clinician assumes that narcissistic people are incapable of altruism. Many of us are prone to regard narcissism and altruism as being at opposite ends of a continuum, but in fact, some people with serious narcissistic psychopathology are also capable of being generous with their time and energy in the service of helping others. Many physicians and clergy, for example, are highly devoted to their patients or parishioners because they derive narcissistic gratification from helping others. Whether that amounts to healthy narcissism or some form of pathological narcissism is often difficult to determine.

An overarching consideration in this context is that in most cases, people who are altruistic are directly benefiting from their altruism (Gabbard and Crisp-Han 2016). If a stranger sees a child who has fallen into a roaring river, he or she may rescue the child not only for altruistic reasons but also to receive acclaim as a hero in the local news media. In fact, in a neuroimaging study, Moll et al. (2006) demonstrated how altruistic behaviors are directly beneficial to the person who is performing such behaviors. Participants in the study had to choose to endorse or oppose societal causes by anonymous decisions to donate or refrain from donating to real charitable organizations. The mesolimbic reward system was engaged when participants *donated* money in the same way as it was when they *received* monetary awards. The investigators inferred that altruism activates brain centers that are associated with selfish pleasures like sex or eating.

The capacity to work and love is often viewed as a sign of mental health, but the situation is more complex when clinicians look for narcissistic pathology. Many narcissists are able to perform at high levels in their chosen profession. A better reflection of their health or pathology is to examine the range of relationships and their quality. A useful diagnostic tool is to encourage the patient to characterize how she regards herself and others and listen with a nonjudgmental ear.

Narcissism has its own developmental course along a continuum from primitive to healthy or mature. Moreover, there are regressions in this developmental pathway—for example, midlife passage, aging, and the specter of death—that make it difficult to consider whether narcissism is pathological or healthy in any one moment of time. Context must be taken into account. Poland (2017) notes that healthy or mature narcissism "serves the self by cherishing the other, by caring about others and about ideals beyond oneself" (p. 97). Individuals with pathological narcissism struggle with trying to obtain the response they need from others in order to maintain a sense of self-esteem. Those with mature narcissism have some degree of resilience in the face of narcissistic injury and can bounce back from a blow. Yet these distinctions may become blurred when self-doubt is activated.

There is also confusion about whether narcissistic patients genuinely feel distress or simply stir up distress in others. Clinicians often tend to minimize the emotional pain that narcissistic patients feel. In a rigorous study of a nationally representative sample of 34,365 individuals, Eaton et al. (2017) investigated how NPD related to other mental disorders using the model of internalizing versus externalizing factors to determine how these dimensions applied to NPDs. The internalizing factors had two subfactors: distress and fear, typical of anxiety disorder and mood disorders. Externalizing factors typical of antisocial personality disorder, borderline personality disorder, and substance abuse were also considered. The results indicated that NPD was best conceptualized as a disorder of distress for both men and women. It is highly possible that this high level of distress may be obscured by the grandiosity and self-promotion of many narcissists as well as by the therapist's feeling of distress in trying to engage the patient in a collaborative process.

Identifying who is narcissistic and who is not is far too "all or none" for the complex understanding required. Different narcissistic persons have different ways of relating. Because of the variations seen in the way that narcissists treat others, a careful examination of modes of relatedness is crucial in trying to gain a greater understanding of the idiosyncratic aspects of each narcissistic patient. In Chapter 3, "Modes of Relatedness," we discuss these variations in detail.

THE NARCISSISTIC CONTINUUM

Yet another diagnostic dilemma encountered by clinicians is the *severity* of the narcissistic features. Caligor et al. (2015) pointed out that of all the personality disorders, the broadest spectrum of severity occurs in NPD. This distinction may be particularly relevant in assessing the degree of antisocial or psychopathic behavior in a patient. Narcissistic disturbances are often conceptualized on a continuum with psychopathy (Gabbard 2014; Kernberg 2014). The reader must keep in mind that positions on a hypothetical continuum are not reified or rigid and can shift on the basis of the emotional or interpersonal context.

Mild narcissistic problems falling short of true NPD appear at the highest level of the continuum, and psychopathy is at the lowest level. True psychopaths are totally incapable of investing themselves in nonexploitative relationships and cannot conceive of others as having altruistic motives. Approximately 20%–50% of those who meet criteria for antisocial personality disorder also meet the criteria for psychopathy (Hare 2006). Psychopathy appears to have significant biological origins, as suggested by studies of children with callous-unemotional traits, including such characteristics as total lack of empathy and an absence of guilt (Blair et al. 2001). Such children cannot process fear and sadness.

They may also have less amygdalar reactivity to fearful faces compared with other children of the same age (Jones et al. 2009). Thus, psychopaths may appear to be narcissistic in the way they relate to others, but the disturbance is far more profound and inalterable than those narcissistic personalities at the higher levels of the continuum.

One can differentiate antisocial personality disorder proper from true psychopathy by the existence of some capacity for anxiety and depression, which reflects the existence of superego components. Hence, a key part of an assessment on this spectrum is to look for deficits in the patient's superego, a pattern of dishonesty, and a callous attitude toward hurting others. The exact point at which antisocial personality disorder transitions into NPD is difficult to pinpoint. Kernberg (1998) suggests that malignant narcissism resides one step up on the continuum from antisocial personality disorder. This entity is characterized by ego-syntonic sadism and a paranoid orientation. These individuals differ from psychopathic and antisocial individuals in that they have some capacity for loyalty and concern for others. They can also imagine that other people may have moral concerns and convictions. This capacity is not present in the true psychopath, who assumes that in every encounter the other person is operating only out of self-interest.

One step up from the malignant narcissist is NPD, with some degree of antisocial behavior. Individuals with NPD lack the sadistic and paranoid qualities of the malignant narcissist but nevertheless may be capable of exploiting others in the service of their own goals. However, they do experience guilt and concern for others and can plan realistically for the future. Their difficulty in making a commitment to in-depth relationships may be reflected in what appears to be antisocial behavior.

At the higher end of the narcissistic continuum, clinicians see many patients who are not a "pure culture" of NPD. They have idiosyncratic mixtures of characterological features that are interwoven. Those who fit the category of the high-functioning subtype may be professionals who have achieved considerable acclaim in their fields. Many of them have obsessive-compulsive features and are workaholics. Perfectionism is a core feature of obsessive-compulsive personality disorder, and Rothstein (1980) has identified the pursuit of perfection as a significant feature of pathological narcissism. This combination of narcissistic and obsessive-compulsive features may lead to overbearing and controlling behavior with others, but people with this mixed characterological picture may also be capable of empathizing with others and having reciprocity and mutuality in relationships. Although they may joke about their compulsiveness, they rarely make light of their narcissism. Most prefer to consider their driven behavior as having its origins in obsessive-compulsive tendencies.

The use of diagnostic labels is also affected by gender stereotyping. When one uses the term "narcissist," listeners may automatically think that a male is being referred to. On the other hand, if one uses the term "histrionic," the stereotype of an emotionally volatile and highly seductive woman may enter one's mind—a modern day version of Scarlett O'Hara. Similarly, borderline personality disorder is far more common in females than in males, and some narcissistic females are diagnosed as having borderline personality disorder. As Kernberg (1975) has long stressed, someone who meets criteria for NPD may well have an underlying borderline personality organization.

The assumption that men are more likely to be narcissistic than women does not hold up to scrutiny. Klonsky et al. (2002) conducted an empirical study of 665 college students and found that the study subjects who behaved in a way that was an exaggerated version of their gender exhibited more narcissistic features, regardless of whether they were male or female. The authors speculated that there may be masculine and feminine ways of being narcissistic that reflect gender stereotypes within the culture.

Those individuals who have some mixture of histrionic/hysterical personality and narcissistic personality traits may present considerable diagnostic complexity. Many histrionic persons can seem vain and exhibitionistic in the way that some narcissistic persons are. It may be highly challenging to determine if there is a greater capacity to care about others and to empathize with the feelings of others. Variations of these combinations occur, so it is often necessary to continually assess the level of severity as the evaluation or treatment goes forward.

Obviously, there can be considerable overlap between borderline and narcissistic personality features as well. However, the narcissistic patient is somewhat more stable and consistent and less likely to engage in highly impulsive and self-destructive behaviors such as self-mutilation. When we attempt to identify features that distinguish NPD from other personality disorders, however, we must keep in mind that research demonstrates that there is significant comorbidity with other personality disorders, particularly histrionic and antisocial, and with passive-aggressive behavior (Clemence et al. 2009).

Another diagnostic quandary appears on the higher end of the narcissistic continuum. Hypervigilant narcissists may present as having avoidant personality disorder or even social anxiety disorder. These patients may be wary of interactions with others for fear of disapproval, criticism, or rejection. They are reluctant to involve themselves with others unless they are assured of being liked. However, avoidant individuals feel inadequate and lack the underlying grandiosity of the hypervigilant narcissist.

Some vulnerable or hypervigilant patients will also present with a clinical picture that involves the interface of masochism and narcissism. Cooper (1993) wrote that one often finds prominent narcissistic traits in a masochistic or self-defeating patient. These individuals go through life as grievance collectors and are always blaming others for their problems. These patients may seem overtly empathic and self-sacrificing, but just underneath the surface it is clear that they are interested primarily in how they have been mistreated and in their own suffering. They often feel they have earned a special distinction in that they have suffered more extensively and more severely than anyone else they know. From their point of view, their extraordinary suffering should be deserving of special recognition by others. When that acknowledgment is not forthcoming, they can feel victimized yet again. A common development in the course of treatment is that patients grow increasingly convinced that the therapist is not empathizing with how they see things but instead is trying to help the patient see a spouse's or partner's point of view. They may then become righteously indignant and may terminate their treatment abruptly. They may ultimately see a string of therapists, each of whom fails them—in the patients' view—by "blaming" them for their own suffering.

Self-defeating trends are pervasive in narcissistic patients. Indeed, one of the tragic features that is present in virtually all narcissistic patients is that they undermine the affirming, admiring response from others that they desperately seek. The more they try to control how others should react to them, the more they alienate those whom they wish to impress. Their neediness is too much for most people. Moreover, once they get close to someone, they may feel worse because the other person has qualities that they lack. Another tragic dimension is that they are so busy trying to achieve, excel, attract attention, be the "star," and otherwise upstage their perceived rivals that they are likely to miss their lives. In other words, they find it difficult to have the day-to-day gratifications that bring meaning to one's life. Their quest for perfection leaves them always falling short and rarely satisfied.

DIAGNOSING NARCISSISM IN AN ERA OF INTERSUBJECTIVITY

Psychoanalytic thinking has evolved beyond a one-person psychology in the past few decades such that the intersubjectivity of any therapeutic dyad is a given. In other words, each member of the dyad enters the relationship with an internalized family system and an idiosyncratic self-structure that has emerged from an imperfect past. With all their baggage in tow, the two partners in the enterprise then jointly create the atmosphere of the therapy. Clinicians have their own struggles with maintaining self-esteem, and a narcissistic desire to do well with the patient can be the battlefield on which that struggle is enacted. Many of the great innovators in psychoanalysis, including Freud himself, are said to have been narcissistic. In fact, that particular adjective is a favorite weapon used by one clinician against another who seems to be more successful or admired. Moreover, as clinicians, we may have blind spots with narcissistic patients when they have a form of narcissism that cuts too close to the bone for us. It is easy to projectively disavow our own self-esteem issues and see them only in the patient. In contemporary discourse, the narcissist has become the "other"—someone "not like me." Yet some high-functioning narcissists may also charm and impress the therapist to the point that diagnostic blind spots are created. The assessor may feel "special" because of the flattery of the narcissistic patient who has come for help.

The complexity of narcissistic psychopathology is daunting. It is probably in the best interest of the patient and, for that matter, the ultimate treatment, if the clinician does not reductively focus on whether the patient does or does not have NPD. Such an approach is excessively binary and likely to lead to misunderstandings. Most of us have the wish to do well in life and be respected by others. We all have some degree of narcissism, and it reveals itself in particular contexts that have special meanings to us. Our vulnerabilities become apparent when triggers in the present activate old wounds from the past. Indeed, it is precisely our own capacity for narcissistic desires and injuries that allows us to empathize and identify with the suffering of the narcissistic patient. A far more useful approach to diagnosis and treatment is to avoid obsessing about whether the patient meets particular criteria and instead assess the narcissistic themes in the material as they emerge and see how they interface with other traits to create a unique person. After all, Hippocrates taught us that knowing the diagnosis is not as important as knowing who the person with the diagnosis is.

REFERENCES

Ackerman RA, Hands AJ, Donnellan MB, et al: Experts' views regarding the conceptualization of narcissism. J Pers Disord 31(3):346–361, 2017 27322575

American Psychiatric Association: Diagnostic and Statistical Manual of Mental Disorders, 4th Edition. Washington, DC, American Psychiatric Association, 1994

American Psychiatric Association: Diagnostic and Statistical Manual of Mental Disorders, 5th Edition. Arlington, VA, American Psychiatric Association, 2013

Beharry WT: Disarming the Narcissist, 2nd Edition. Oakland, CA, New Harbinger, 2013

Blair RJ, Colledge E, Murray L, et al: A selective impairment in the processing of sad and fearful expressions in children with psychopathic tendencies. J Abnorm Child Psychol 29(6):491–498, 2001 11761283

Burgo J: The Narcissist You Know: Defending Yourself Against Extreme Narcissists in an All-About-Me Age, New York, Touchstone, 2015

Caligor E, Levy KN, Yeomans FE: Narcissistic personality disorder: diagnostic and clinical challenges. Am J Psychiatry 172(5):415–422, 2015 25930131

Campbell WK, Miller JD (eds): The Handbook of Narcissism and Narcissistic Personality Disorder: Theoretical Approaches, Empirical Findings, and Treatments. Hoboken, NJ, Wiley, 2011

Carlson EN, Oltmanns TF: The role of metaperception in personality disorders: do people with personality problems know how others experience their personality? J Pers Disord 29(4):449–467, 2015 26200846

Clemence AJ, Perry JC, Plakun EM: Narcissistic and borderline personality disorders in a sample of treatment refractory patients. Psychiatr Ann 39(4):175–184, 2009

Cooper AM: Psychotherapeutic approaches to masochism. J Psychother Pract Res 2(1):51–63, 1993 22700126

Dickinson KA, Pincus AL: Interpersonal analysis of grandiose and vulnerable narcissism. J Pers Disord 17(3):188–207, 2003 12839099

Dombek K: The Selfishness of Others: An Essay on the Fear of Narcissism. New York, Farrar, Straus, and Giroux, 2016

Eaton NR, Rodriguez-Seijas C, Krueger RF, et al: Narcissistic personality disorder and the structure of common mental disorders. J Pers Disord 31(4):449–461, 2017 27617650

Gabbard GO: Two subtypes of narcissistic personality disorder. Bull Menninger Clin 53(6):527–532, 1989 2819295

Gabbard GO: Transference and countertransference in the treatment of narcissistic patients, in Disorders of Narcissism: Diagnostic, Clinical and Empirical Implications. Edited by Ronningstam EF. Washington, DC, American Psychiatric Press, 1998, pp 125–146

Gabbard GO: Psychodynamic Psychiatry in Clinical Practice, 5th Edition. Arlington, VA, American Psychiatric Publishing, 2014

Gabbard GO, Crisp-Han H: The many faces of narcissism. World Psychiatry 15(2):115–116, 2016 27265694

Gunderson JG, Hoffman PD (eds): Understanding and Treating Borderline Personality Disorder: A Clinical Guide for Professionals and Families. Arlington, VA, American Psychiatric Publishing, 2005

Hare RD: Psychopathy: a clinical and forensic overview. Psychiatr Clin North Am 29(3):709–724, 2006 16904507

Jones AP, Laurens KR, Herba CM, et al: Amygdala hypoactivity to fearful faces in boys with conduct problems and callous-unemotional traits. Am J Psychiatry 166(1):95–102, 2009 18923070

Kernberg OF: Borderline Conditions and Pathological Narcissism. Northvale, NJ, Aronson, 1975

Kernberg OF: Severe Personality Disorders: Psychotherapeutic Strategies. New Haven, CT, Yale University Press, 1984

Kernberg OF: Pathological narcissism and narcissistic personality disorder: theoretical background and diagnostic classification, in Disorders of Narcissism: Diagnostic, Clinical, and Empirical Implications. Edited by Ronningstam EF, Washington, DC, American Psychiatric Press, 1998, pp 29–51

Kernberg OF: An overview of the treatment of severe narcissistic pathology. Int J Psychoanal 95(5):865–888, 2014 24902768

Klonsky ED, Jane JS, Turkheimer E, et al: Gender role and personality disorders. J Pers Disord 16(5):464–476, 2002 12489312

Kohut H: The Analysis of the Self. Madison, WI, International Universities Press, 1971

Kohut H: The Restoration of the Self. New York, International Universities Press, 1977

Moll J, Krueger F, Zahn R, et al: Human fronto-mesolimbic networks guide decisions about charitable donation. Proc Natl Acad Sci USA 103(42):15,623–15,628, 2006 17030808

Pincus AL, Lukowitsky MR: Pathological narcissism and narcissistic personality disorder. Annu Rev Clin Psychol 6:421–446, 2010 20001728

Poland W: Intimacy and Separateness in Psychoanalysis. Oxford, UK, Routledge, 2017

Rosenfeld H: Impasse and Interpretation: Therapeutic and Anti-Therapeutic Factors in the Psychoanalytic Treatment of Psychotic, Borderline, and Neurotic Patients. London, Tavistock, 1987

Rothstein A: The Narcissistic Pursuit of Perfection. New York, International Universities Press, 1980

Russ E, Shedler J, Bradley R, et al: Refining the construct of narcissistic personality disorder: diagnostic criteria and subtypes. Am J Psychiatry 165(11):1473–1481, 2008 18708489

Skodol AE, Bender DS, Morey LC, et al: Personality disorder types proposed for DSM-5. J Pers Disord 25(2):136–169, 2011 21466247

Steiner J: Seeing and being seen: narcissistic pride and narcissistic humiliation. Int J Psychoanal 87(Pt 4):939–951, 2006 16877245

Wink P: Two faces of narcissism. J Pers Soc Psychol 61(4):590–597, 1991 1960651

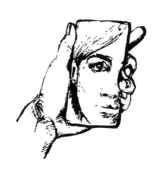

2

The Cultural Context of Narcissism

In 1979, Christopher Lasch came out with an extraordinarily popular book, *The Culture of Narcissism*, in which he made a persuasive argument that the electronic media thrives on superficial images, which leads to shallowness and lack of depth in the lives of many American citizens (Lasch 1979). Television, advertising, and popular movies are replete with handsome and beautiful people with perfect bodies, white teeth, and flowing hair. Their clothes, of course, are impeccable. Words, ideas, and thoughtful perspectives have become irrelevant. Billy Crystal's character Fernando on *Saturday Night Live* captured it in a pithy statement: "It is not how you feel, it is how you look!"

Thirty years after the publication of Lasch's book, Twenge and Campbell (2009) wrote *The Narcissism Epidemic*. Unlike Lasch, whose conclusions were impressionistic, these authors drew on a growing body of research about narcissists. Moreover, they focused more attention on the impact of living one's life on social media, the change in parenting styles, and the impact of the ubiquitous handheld phone. Their research has resulted in the concept of *generational narcissism*, as Twenge suggested in the revised edition of *Generation Me* (Twenge 2014). In her view, people born after 1982 are prone to embracing a common set of values that includes a sense of entitlement. For example, these young adults tend to feel that they deserve wealth and fame without having done what is necessary to earn it. A decade ago, the National Institutes of Health sponsored a study of narcissistic personality disorder (NPD; Stinson et al. 2008) that found that there were nearly three times more persons meeting criteria for NPD in the age group from 20 to 29 than in the age group over 65. The millennial generation has grown up with a quantitative means of self-esteem enhancement: the number of "likes" on social media that offer instant gratification throughout the day and into the wee hours of the night. However, millennials are not the only generation affected by the transformative cultural shifts of smartphones and social media—anyone with a device in their pocket is being shaped by the ability to have their needs met on demand, whether with products delivered to the doorstep in under an hour or with texts or posts requiring immediate response.

Twenge and Campbell (2009) noted that in their work they primarily concentrated on the prevalence of narcissistic personality traits within the normal population, recognizing that many of these cases are not sufficiently destructive to the individual and others to warrant the diagnosis of NPD. They saw the major influences on this cultural phenomenon as growing out of more permissive parenting and self-esteem–focused education, a media culture of shallow celebrity, and the widespread prevalence of Internet communication. They also noted that the availability of easy credit can make a reality out of narcissistic dreams without people thinking much about future consequences. These factors have led to a culture in which people mistake extreme narcissism for solid self-esteem. The two are actually quite different.

Self-admiration is a key feature of this cultural narcissism. The selfie phenomenon is pervasive among young people, who must be the most video-recorded and photographed generation ever. Parents now experience grade school or middle school functions as a fight with other parents to secure the best possible location to photograph their children in the act of reciting, dancing, singing, or playing a musical instrument. Extraordinary numbers of handheld phones and camcorders end up blocking the views of other parents trying to take similar pictures.

From another perspective, one might argue that the smartphone is essentially taking over the parental function in that it provides a way through which people can represent themselves. One could compare this phenomenon to the way that taking photographs of works of art alters the experience of the original artwork itself (P. Ringstrom, personal communication, August 2017). There is an unacknowledged tragic dimension to this effort to capture the moment in a smartphone video or photo: In distancing oneself from the immediate experience, there is a risk of missing the precious moments of one's life.

It is common for some young people to become focused on presenting themselves in the best light by taking 100 selfies at a time and spending an hour or two narrowing the number down to 5. They agonize over selecting the final choice, one that will present them in the most stunning possible way. Before the chosen picture is posted, it may be photoshopped to enhance the individual's figure or physique.

> A 26-year-old junior executive in the energy business spent most of Sunday afternoon obsessing about which bikini-clad photo would make her the most irresistible. After her selection of the photo, she worked meticulously to improve it by photoshopping her picture to make her hair blonder and her figure thinner. She waited until the following day, Monday, to post the photo during the noon hour, knowing that Monday through Friday between the hours of noon and 3 P.M. are high-traffic times when one will get the most responses. When she finally posted it, she played it down with the accompanying understated description: "Enjoying this beautiful weather." This same patient told her therapist that she was concerned about how social media is affecting dating. She complained that "Singles don't want to 'hook up' unless they've first seen a nude photo. I suppose it prevents a lot of wasted time, but I'm not sure I want to go there."

Facebook and other social media sites have also become the preferred way of hurting someone in the peer group. By commenting on everyone else's posts but selectively *not* commenting on those of a particular individual, one can inflict narcissistic wounds to the neglected victim. The injured party may then stalk those who declined to comment to see if they were traveling or otherwise indisposed around the time of the post. If not, the wound may be even deeper. Narcissism is taking over social media. How many followers or friends one has on social media has become far more important than how much money one earns, what kind of car one owns, or the status of one's job. In the view of people today, there is no better self-validation than to boast about how many people are interested in your every move. However, false advertising is another outgrowth of the narcissistic vulnerability that goes with social media. A favorite birthday card illustrates this phenomenon: "May your life someday be as awesome as you pretend it is on Facebook."

The young people who are growing up in Generation Me often feel cheated. They feel they were raised to be special, but they have not been able to achieve what their parents led them to believe was possible. Some millennials blame their baby boomer parents for their plight (Twenge 2014). Baby boomers, on the other hand, often complain about the poorly developed work ethic of young people and their assumption that they should receive high pay and generous time off simply because of who they are. Bosses often complain that when a young employee is asked to do something, a common answer is "Why?" The response from the boss to that query may well be "Because I told you to," a response not well received by the youthful employee.

Twenge and Campbell (2009) recognized that many of the narcissists they describe in the millennial group are not true NPDs but rather individuals who have high levels of narcissism and think they are better than others even when they are not. These narcissists generally lack warm, caring, and loving relationships and in many cases feel superior to others. They are generally regarded as self-serving and have a tendency to live life online so that others can observe their accomplishments, their love lives, and their thoughts and feelings. In their research, Twenge and Campbell used the Narcissistic Personality Inventory (NPI), and they acknowledge that most people above the 90th percentile of the NPI scale do not have diagnosable clinical NPD according to the DSM-5 criteria (American Psychiatric Association 2013).

Perhaps the most often cited characteristic of the generational narcissists is that they feel *entitled*. They may think, for example, that they should be paid a $200,000 salary to sit in a room and design video games. They think they are entitled to leave work whenever they wish to, play basketball or video games during breaks, have free snacks available to them in the office, and do whatever they want when they want. However, entitlement alone is not indicative of severe narcissistic pathology. In fact, research on entitlement (Crowe et al. 2016) suggests that there is considerable heterogeneity among individuals who feel entitled. Although these individuals generally fall into two groups, one emotionally stable and the other emotionally vulnerable, the studies do not establish criteria that make the cluster differences theoretically or clinically meaningful. Like narcissism itself, entitlement occurs on a spectrum and manifests itself in different ways with different individuals.

Twenge and Campbell (2009) also recognized that there is a significant difference between narcissism as it manifests in an individual patient coming to a mental health professional for treatment and narcissism as a cultural phenomenon. They note that what they view as a narcissism epidemic involves two intertwining stories. One of those stories involves individuals with high levels of narcissism, whereas the other reflects a shift in our shared cultural values toward greater narcissism and self-admiration.

In their work, Twenge (2014) and Twenge and Campbell (2009) stressed that the narcissists they focused on in their research about the Me Generation are much more in keeping with the grandiose extroverted individual rather than the hypervigilant narcissist who is feeling slighted at every turn. There is some overlap between the clinical population and the cultural trend among the millennial population, but it is easy to forget that there are major differences. The NPI measures variations of normal or healthy narcissism, and all the data gathered are from self-report.

Some critics have questioned the Generation Me categorization because of the greater altruism of twenty-somethings. Arnett (2013) argued that they are more conscious of their relation to others, more empathic, and more generous than generations before them. In fact, millennials tend to be better at connecting with one another and expecting to be helped by others while providing help to those who need it as well. They also may be more socially conscious. Moreover, they are dedicated to service projects, are socially aware, and contribute to charity at a higher rate than do their elders (Kristof 2015). Hence, many observers take issue with the sweeping statements being made about an entire generation, knowing that the generalizations apply to some individuals and not to others. Psychodynamic and psychoanalytic understanding and treatment are geared to what is unique and idiosyncratic about the individual rather than broad cultural trends. Of course, a psychoanalyst or psychotherapist is not blind to cultural influences, but nevertheless, persons in these professions tend to keep in mind how the individual tends to vary from cultural stereotypes.

One of the major differences between psychological research on the one hand and the clinical accounts of narcissistic patients (Caligor et al. 2015; Gabbard 1998, 2013; Kealy et al. 2015; Kernberg 2014) on the other lies in the fact that individual patients are seen in therapy sessions over time. The data gathered by a clinician longitudinally is a different category of observation than a survey at a point in time. Some researchers have concluded from self-report questionnaires that narcissism is what it appears to be—overly high self-esteem. In other words, these individuals really think that they are better than others and like to talk about it. In this view, their presentation is not a defensive strategy motivated by unconscious factors. Clinicians, on the other hand, have a different view. On the basis of long-term psychoanalytic psychotherapy, they see that these patients are often terribly insecure under the surface. In fact, the person who brags the longest and loudest is likely to be the most worried about his or her self-worth underneath. Psychotherapy often reveals that there is an emptiness in NPD patients and a feeling that they do not have a clear sense of self. Those who may appear grandiose can be shattered by a slight or criticism and appear to fall apart in narcissistic rage or despair. Clinicians are reluctant to take the self-confidence of an arrogant, grandiose individual at face value. They know that these patients are not impervious to a blow to their self-esteem.

In light of the fact that Twenge (2014) acknowledged that in the vast majority of cases, the millennials studied do not cross the threshold of DSM-5 NPD, we would certainly expect there to be differences between college students and those persons seen in a clinical context. Moreover, we must keep in mind that overindulgent parenting styles, such as "helicopter parenting," have played a major role in the sense of entitlement of this generation.

A mother and her 17-year-old daughter were seen together in a clinical consultation because the daughter was rebelling against her mother, and the following exchange ensued.

> **Mother:** If you don't get into one of the four colleges your father and I have suggested, you are going to regret it the rest of your life. If you go to a crappy college, you will face a life filled with crappy jobs!
> **Daughter:** I don't care! I'm different than you and Dad. Can't you see that?
> **Mother:** You don't understand. We are trying to help you see that decisions you make now will affect you the rest of your life. Can't you see we are doing all of this for *you?*
> **Daughter:** Don't give me that bullshit! You aren't doing this for me— you want me to get into Stanford for *you!* Then you can brag about me and have everyone in the neighborhood think that you must be wonderful parents!
> **Mother:** No, Honey. Everything we are doing is for you, not me. That hurts my feelings.

Some young people will say that they feel entitled because their parents made them that way. Hence, they may feel a limited sense of agency. Rebellion may be their way of creating an identity of their own apart from their parents. Those who *do* follow the path prescribed by their parents may feel they are never doing enough and may harbor a chronic sense of shame about falling short of parental expectations.

It is important to note that more recent data derived from Twenge's research point to a new generation, which she calls *iGen*, the generation subsequent to the millennials who have come of age since the advent of the iPhone in 2007. Her observations note a serious trend—a seismic increase not in narcissism but in anxiety and depression in children and teens who have grown up with the constant comparisons to others that social media creates (Twenge 2017). This research suggests there is a darker side to the culture of living online with pervasive social media access.

LIVING IN CYBERSPACE

There can be little doubt that the Internet has had more profound changes in the way we live our lives in the past few decades than has any other influence. Narcissism is fundamentally about difficulties regarding how we see self and other and how we relate to one another. The Internet has contributed to these dimensions of existence in far-reaching ways. Posting what one is doing—and what a great time one is having while doing it—seems to be more significant than actually savoring what one is doing by living authentically in the moment.

A young woman who broke up with her boyfriend came to therapy wondering what she should do. As the patient continued to talk, it became clear to the therapist that "What should I do?" applied more to how she should present herself on social media to her hundreds of "friends" rather than how she should deal psychologically with the breakup. She knew she had to change her status, but she was terribly concerned about how others might see her. The image she conveyed to others was clearly much more important than some form of genuine grieving in real time.

There is something inherently narcissistic about social media such as Facebook, Snapchat, and Instagram (Chandra 2017). Many people can observe one's success, and one can shape what the "audience" sees to enhance the positive elements. Indeed, young adults who spend much of their time on social media often feel that they must sacrifice authenticity to be appealing. When meeting someone through a dating app, they may feel it is necessary to keep up the "enhanced" image of themselves to the person they are dating, even if it means being dishonest. Raw data from Google searches demonstrate that we are not who we seem to be on social media (Stephens-Davidowitz 2017). There is a "surface" quality to social media communications that may be a good fit with narcissistically organized participants. But there is a "chicken or the egg" dilemma with social media—does social media make those who use it narcissistic, or were they like that in the first place and simply are attracted to this form of communication? There is some research suggesting that a higher level of narcissism predicts more time on Facebook (Buffardi and Campbell 2008). Chandra (2017) also points out that narcissistic people may spend more time on Facebook, so a relatively small population is overrepresented online.

Research shows that selfies are perceived to be more narcissistic, less trustworthy, and less socially attractive to people who view them (Kramer et al. 2017). In other words, some people may use social media as a way of saying to the world, "Look at me! Please notice me!" Chandra (2017) suggested that social media in general is an engine of narcissism. If narcissism was not present in an individual before that person gets hooked on social media, it may be afterward.

The indispensable vehicle of the selfie is, of course, the handheld device that is called a phone but often is purchased primarily for its many other uses. When we go to a party, a conference, or a gathering of colleagues, we note that for the most part, each individual is absorbed in cyberspace communication on his or her smartphone more than in face-to-face contact with real individuals in the environment. Sherry Turkle, a professor at the Massachusetts Institute of Technology who has been a diligent student of the contemporary problems related to the fact that we live our lives in the digital world, describes this as "there but not there" (Turkle 2011, p. 14). In her research she has noted that most of us are concerned about whether we are closer together or farther apart, and monitoring this level of relatedness consumes us. She quotes the 13-year-old who tells her that she cannot stand using the phone and never listens to voice mail, but texting offers exactly the right amount of control and distance. A 21-year-old college student views phone calls as too time consuming. She can gather what she needs to know from someone's Facebook wall, Twitter, and texting. Turkle (2011) describes the situation as follows: "I once described a computer as a second self, a mirror of mind. Now the metaphor no longer goes far enough. Our new devices provide space for the emergence of a new state of the self, itself split between the screen and the physically real, wired into existence through technology" (p. 16). Over time, online life is becoming life itself.

The age of the ubiquitous smartphone has contributed substantially to the narcissism of contemporary culture. While two people are chatting at dinner, one or both make recurrent glances at their mobile devices, clarifying that they are only partially present for their dinner companion. Conferences now feature one person speaking while the majority of the audience is doing their best to listen to the speech, at least partially, while simultaneously attending to texts and e-mails. Most of us think we do rather well at multitasking, but in reality, we are recognizing that our bodies are rewarding us with neurochemicals that induce a multitasking "high." Although we may *think* that we are being especially productive, multitaskers are found in research not to perform as well in any of the tasks they are attempting compared with non-multitaskers (Turkle 2011).

The self traditionally has been shaped by a combination of how others see you and your own reflection on yourself during time alone, when you can attend to private thoughts. Intimacy has generally required privacy, but as Turkle (2011) points out, intimacy without privacy reinvents what we mean by *intimacy.* We are alone together.

The constant bombardment of adolescents and young adults with e-mails, text messages, social media postings, and other forms of cybercommunication has another impact: There is no "time out" to contemplate the developing self amid the flurry of stimuli. The dopamine bursts crowd out reflective time to figure out who one is in a sea of confusing communications from outside. Both D. W. Winnicott (1965) and Erik Erikson (1950) emphasized the need for late adolescents and young adults to have a relatively incommunicado period during which they can look inward and get to know themselves. Focusing intensively on self-development is necessary to balance narcissistic needs with concern for others, and today's youth may have no such opportunity.

The images one contemplates are also misleading and deceptive. As Turkle (2011) noted, the "real me" is unlikely to appear on a Facebook page. As noted earlier in this chapter, it is common for adolescents and young adult females to use software on their profile photographs that allows them to appear thinner or more shapely than they actually are. Indeed, social media itself seem to implore us to represent ourselves in ways that are highly oversimplified.

Turkle (2011) succinctly sums up a situation that has developed as result of living our lives in cyberspace:

> We are connected as we have never been connected before, and we seem to have damaged ourselves in the process. A 2010 analysis of data from over 14,000 college students over the past 30 years shows that since the year 2000, young people have reported a dramatic decline in interest in other people. Today's college students are, for example, far less likely to say that it is valuable to try to put oneself in the place of others or to try to understand their feelings. (p. 293)

It is clear that empathy has fallen as we now field one inauthentic communication after another and try to position ourselves as responding in a way that will present ourselves in a favorable light. Perhaps the most distressing aspect of this cultural shift is how rare it is to find someone who is truly present when in the company of others.

NARCISSISM, LOVE, AND INTIMACY IN A WORLD OF VIRTUAL COMMUNICATION

It is commonplace these days for romances to begin online, often continue online for a period of time, and even end while remaining virtual throughout. In some cases, the lovers never meet, and the image of the beloved is a mixture of the sound of a voice, the language of love, and the fantasy of the partner. The ultimate extension of this form of relationship is a human relating to a machine as a partner. Indeed, in Turkle's (2011) survey of technology and its impact today, she observed that over time, programmers become very attached to their computer, and something of a connection is formed, one she describes as "democratized." One can hardly avoid the conclusion that computers have become our companions. We now have sociable robots and online agents explicitly designed to convince us that they are the kinds of partners that we are looking for. There was even a 2016 conference in London titled "Love and Sex with Robots" (Bendel 2017). Topics dealt with included whether or not the robot should be free to refuse to perform a sex act.

In America, the Hollywood cinema has long been a reflector of the current zeitgeist. Signifiers of the culture are present on the great silver screen in a way that allows audiences to recognize who they are and what they are about in a particular era. In 1998, Tom Hanks and Meg Ryan starred in *You've Got Mail*, a romantic comedy that made the phrase "you've got mail" a universal signifier of connection. The e-mail chats of the two central characters grow into intimate conversations, which in turn blossom into romance. At the end, the lovers meet in Riverside Park, where it becomes clear that they will live happily ever after.

Two decades later, Spike Jonze created *Her*, a world where marrying a virtual spouse seems to be an attractive possibility. In this film, Theodore (Joaquin Phoenix) is mesmerized by the sensual voice of Samantha, an "Individual Operating System" (OS1). Played by actress Scarlett Johansson, Samantha's voice truly weaves a spell over Theodore, who has been melancholy for some time since having been dumped by his ex-wife. He has withdrawn from relationships and spends much of his time with machines, computers, his smartphone, and video games. In the midst of his struggle with deciding if he should sign the divorce papers, Theodore is in dialogue with Samantha, who provides a soothing voice and an inner responsive presence, helping him survive the melancholy crisis of rejection that is his daily life. Samantha's voice is sweet, never angry, always empathic, accommodating to his Theodore's needs, and a veritable ideal love relationship that comes to him with a flick of a switch.

The OS1 that creates Samantha's voice is designed to adapt to Theodore's desires and needs. Samantha appears to know what he wishes to hear before he asks for it. Samantha may present as the ideal woman to Theodore, but the intimacy goes in only one direction. In essence, she is part of a game in which one party manipulates and uses the other (Sabbadini et al. 2017). Samantha represents the idealized narcissistic love object for Theodore, someone who anticipates his every need and lives only to please him. However, he is crushed to learn that Samantha has a love relationship just like this one with 641 of her other clients. He feels hurt, betrayed, and duped.

The film problematizes the fantasy that if only one met the perfect fusional, narcissistic love object who lives for her master, fulfillment would be complete. The woman is under the omnipotent control of the man because he is in charge of the controls, and there is the potential for the relationship to go on and on in such a way that grief and loss will be avoided. The love object becomes a narcissistic extension of the human subject, and the hope is that the negation of the other as a subject will provide the ideal relationship. Indeed, in this regard the film depicts the common disillusionment that occurs in a narcissistic love relationship, in which the beloved object cannot respond perfectly to the whims and desires of the partner. The discovery of the subjectivity of the other is often the beginning of the collapse in a relationship with a narcissistically organized individual. Samantha attempts to become the perfect partner by never asking for anything for herself and never disappointing. Cyborgs may be able to exist in a world without having their own subjectivity, but in flesh and blood relationships, the two subjectivities involved in a love relationship must learn to accommodate each other's needs.

Her is also a commentary on the extensive availability of all forms of pornography on the Internet. The shift from X-rated cinema houses and video stores to the home computer has had a profound impact on this fantasy of the love object who exists only to satisfy the whim of the viewer. For a relatively reasonable fee, anyone can access the specific fantasy that turns them on, unencumbered by any concerns about what a partner may wish and without anxiety that others will see what they are doing. The viewer's particular narrative of desire appears onscreen without any concern whatsoever about the subjectivity and the desires of the partner. The pornographic partner exists only for the pleasure of the other.

Narcissistic themes are central to the films of Spike Jonze. His 1999 film *Being John Malkovich*, which won the Best Picture Award of the National Society of Film Critics, is a hilarious spoof of celebrity narcissism. In the film, a portal in the wall of an office turns out to be an entry into the head of the actor John Malkovich, where one can experience 15 minutes of celebrity in an alternative reality. Those who line up to be John Malkovich for a quarter of an hour discover that a celebrity's life is as ordinary as their own. This riff on Andy Warhol's prediction that in the future everyone will become famous for 15 minutes is a testament to the emptiness of celebrity (Gabbard 2001).

Online culture has fueled a particular form of narcissistic desire that can circumvent the complications of mutuality in real-life relationships and gratify the viewer without having to think about anyone else's needs or wishes. Unbridled narcissism is alive and well in cyberspace. It was perhaps prescient that long ago and far away—in the year 1968—Stanley Kubrick's masterpiece *2001: A Space Odyssey* carried a warning for the future. The computer that assured the safety of the crew, affectionately referred to as HAL, transformed itself into a malevolent force bent on destruction of its human masters. We live in an era when conversations with Alexa and other digital voices may be more common than human-to-human interaction. Social media is eliminating eye-to-eye contact with another person, and texting is diminishing the need for the human voice.

We may think that computers and other forms of artificial intelligence are serving their masters, but the possibility of unforeseen developments must always be considered in our brave new world. When we least expect it, the humanized images on our machines may fail us in ways that we had never imagined.

REFERENCES

American Psychiatric Association: Diagnostic and Statistical Manual of Mental Disorders, 5th Edition. Arlington, VA, American Psychiatric Association, 2013

Arnett JJ: The evidence for Generation We and against Generation Me. Emerging Adulthood 1(1):5–10, 2013

Bendel O: Machine yearning. Harper's Magazine, June 2017, p. 23

Buffardi LE, Campbell WK: Narcissism and social networking Web sites. Pers Soc Psychol Bull 34(10):1303–1314, 2008 18599659

Caligor E, Levy KN, Yeomans FE: Narcissistic personality disorder: diagnostic and clinical challenges. Am J Psychiatry 172(5):415–422, 2015 25930131

Chandra R: Narcissism and Social Media. Presented at American Psychiatric Association Annual Meeting, San Diego, CA, May 2017

Crowe ML, LoPilato AC, Campbell WK, et al: Identifying two groups of entitled individuals: cluster analysis reveals emotional stability and self-esteem distinction. J Pers Disord 30(6):762–775, 2016 26623539

Erikson E: Childhood and Society. New York, WW Norton, 1950

Gabbard GO: Transference and countertransference in the treatment of narcissistic patients, in Disorders of Narcissism: Dagnostic, Clinical, and Empirical Implications. Edited by Ronningstam E. Washington, DC: American Psychiatric Press, 1998, pp 125–146

Gabbard GO: Fifteen minutes of fame revisited: Being John Malkovich. Int J Psychoanal 82(1):177–179, 2001

Gabbard GO: Countertransference issues in the treatment of pathological narcissism, in Understanding and Treating Pathological Narcissism. Edited by Ogrodniczuk JS. Washington, DC, American Psychological Association, 2013, pp 207–218

Kealy D, Ogrodniczuk JS, Joyce AS, et al: Narcissism and relational representations among psychiatric outpatients. J Pers Disord 29(3):393–407, 2015 23398104

Kernberg OF: An overview of the treatment of severe narcissistic pathology. Int J Psychoanal 95(5):865–888, 2014 24902768

Kramer NC, Feurstein M, Kluck JP, et al: Beware of selfies: the impact of photo type on impression formation based on social networking profiles. Front Psychol 8:188, 2017, 28261129

Kristof N: A millennial named Bush. New York Times, July 16, 2015, p. 9

Lasch C: The Culture of Narcissism: American Life in an Age of Diminishing Expectations. New York, WW Norton, 1979

Sabbadini A, Kogan I, Golinelli T (eds): Virtual Intimacy: A Psychoanalytic Lens on Jonze's Her and Other Films. London, Routledge, 2017

Stephens-Davidowitz S: Don't let Facebook make you miserable. New York Times Review section, May 7, 2017, p. 8

Stinson FS, Dawson DA, Goldstein RB, et al: Prevalence, correlates, disability, and comorbidity of DSM-IV narcissistic personality disorder: results from the wave 2 national epidemiologic survey on alcohol and related conditions. J Clin Psychiatry 69(7):1033–1045, 2008 18557663

Turkle S: Alone Together: Why We Expect More from Technology and Less from Each Other. New York, Basic Books, 2011

Twenge JM: Generation Me. New York. Atria, 2014

Twenge JM: Have smartphones destroyed a generation? The Atlantic, September 2017. Available at: www.theatlantic.com/magazine/archive/2017/09/has-the-smartphone-destroyed-a-generation/534198. Accessed August 3, 2017.

Twenge JM, Campbell WK: The Narcissism Epidemic. New York, Atria, 2009

Winnicott DW: Communicating and not communicating leading to a study of certain opposites, in The Maturational Processes and the Facilitating Environment: Studies in the Theory of Emotional Development. New York, International Universities Press, 1965, pp 37–55

3

Modes of Relatedness

As we noted in Chapter 1, "Narcissism and Its Discontents," diagnosing those who are afflicted with narcissistic disturbances can be highly challenging. Some individuals do not appear to be distressed about their situation, whereas others are suffering to the point where family, friends, and colleagues can hardly stand to be around them. Probably the most useful way to approach the diagnostic dilemmas that one encounters is to investigate characteristic modes of relatedness that the patient describes or enacts. A careful examination of the relational patterns reveals valuable information about both the self-structure of the narcissistic patient and the way that self tends to interact with others.

One useful starting point is the capacity of the individual to love. A central problem in someone with pathological narcissism is how to sustain love in a relationship over time. A common presentation is an intense infatuation followed by a rapid breakup when the partner brings up the inevitable and critiques and disappointments occur. The narcissist is more interested in the honeymoon than the marriage. Having said that, however, whether or not a narcissistically disturbed person is truly searching for love is difficult to discern. Validation or adoration may be of greater interest. In addition, partners who lend themselves to easy idealization may fulfill the need of the narcissist to be in the shadow of an idealized other. The typical problems are much broader than a thwarted search for love—they involve complex efforts to relate to others that repeatedly fail the narcissist.

These efforts are manifested in the workplace as well. A narcissistically organized individual in the office may be desperate for acclaim, respect, and admiration from his colleagues and superiors while at the same time believing that certain tasks are beneath him. His feeling of entitlement may actually undermine the responses he seeks. Moreover, the narcissist may bask in the glow of a promotion only to lapse into boredom and disengagement when the hard work begins. The difference between being courted for a new job or promotion and the humdrum routine of the work itself is analogous to the difference between the honeymoon and the marriage. Those who work at the narcissist's side may recoil from his self-absorption, leaving him with a feeling of isolation. Hence, by focusing on the individual's modes of relatedness, the clinician is likely to find the diagnostic clues to the presence of narcissistic personality disorder (NPD) or variants thereof (Gabbard 2014).

Ogrodniczuk and Kealy (2013) noted that "Narcissistic individuals are not necessarily identified by how they feel, but according to how they make others feel" (p. 114). Paradoxically, the narcissistic way of relating to others tends to drive others away, thus undermining narcissists' hope of eliciting the specific responses they need from other people. Their difficulty in regulating self-esteem is both a response to the reaction of others and a cause of that reaction in others. One could say that at the core of the narcissist's being is a sense of futility—he simply cannot control the responses of others that he desperately needs to stabilize his own self-regard.

COMMON MODES OF RELATEDNESS IN NARCISSISTIC PATIENTS

To some extent, the way that narcissistic patients relate to others can be linked to the three empirically observed categories of grandiose, vulnerable, and high functioning reported by Russ et al. (2008). However, these distinctions are not rigid constructs. Rather, they have permeable borders based on context. Particular triggers and interpersonal situations can cause high degrees of fluctuations between vulnerable and grandiose states, and these states are best regarded as fluid rather than fixed (Gabbard 2014; Kealy et al. 2015; Pincus and Lukowitsky 2010; Ronningstam 2011). What all narcissistic characterological configurations have in common is difficulties in both self-regulation and self-esteem. The following list of modes of relatedness is derived from our own clinical experience as well as relevant published research.

A need to elicit admiration, empathy, and validation from the other. To gain this reaction in a conversation with someone else, narcissistic individuals may use many self-references, drop well-known names, and place themselves in favorable light compared with others. In the case of grandiose narcissists, the speaker may appear oblivious to the responses on the listener's face and may show no interest in what anyone else has to say about the matter. This version of relating is perhaps the most common way the term *narcissistic* is used in nonclinical settings, and it may prompt a comment such as the speaker has "a sender but no receiver." In the case of the vulnerable or hypervigilant narcissist, the speaker's attention may be riveted to the listener's face, trying to capture the "gleam in mother's eye" described by Kohut (1971). The other reason to scrutinize the listener's facial expressions is to detect any kind of slight, whether it be inattention, contempt, disagreement, or boredom (Gabbard 1989).

Pseudo self-sufficiency. This style of relatedness, coined by Kernberg (1970), refers to a denial of dependency and an inability to accept help from others. The narcissist may want others to think of him or her as independent, focused, and on top of all situations. This style generally leads the narcissistic individual to feel more isolated and desperate for attention from others.

Denial or prevention of the other's autonomy. People in a relationship with a narcissistic person often feel controlled. Indeed, the continued attention of the narcissistic partner may depend on the other's submission to omnipotent control. This type of domineering behavior is, of course, completely unempathic to the needs of those who are on the receiving end of it. Dickinson and Pincus (2003) and Ogrodniczuk et al. (2009) have linked this need for dominance and control to the grandiose subtype of narcissistic personality. This dimension often emerges in the bedroom when the narcissist professes his needs without regard to the other person's autonomy. Sex becomes a power struggle in which mutuality disappears. A co-created dynamic may occur in which the narcissist finds himself faced with a partner who has become aggressively disengaged in the face of his demands. In this situation, the narcissist's push for his needs to be met actually makes it less likely that his partner will attend to those needs.

Proneness to feeling shame and humiliation in response to relatively mild slights. Narcissistic patients are easily wounded by those who do not agree with them, those who ignore them, or those who criticize them or ridicule them in any way. Shame is a phenomenon in which the individual feels she has fallen short of her grandiose ideal of who she is or what she should be. Shame generally involves an element of exposure as well, so there is a sense of humiliation associated with the slight. In other words, because one or more persons has observed the slight, the narcissistic individual feels as if her inadequacies are exposed to all. Rage and vindictiveness can be a part of this response to being narcissistically wounded on top of the shame and humiliation (Ogrodniczuk and Kealy 2013).

Denial of pain or conflict associated with a turning away from reality. The intense shame and humiliation found in narcissistic disturbances are sometimes avoided by a massive denial of the reality of the specific situation and the pain or conflict that might arise from it. This maneuver can simply involve a pathological inattention to what others are saying or how others are reacting. Many oblivious narcissists will talk "at" someone rather than "to" someone to assure that they do not see any shred of disagreement or contempt in the listener. Some make only minimal eye contact and appear to be talking to anyone in earshot. Still others may experience a disappointment but immediately transform it into a positive turn of events. For example, a man came to therapy and told his therapist he had just been dumped by his girlfriend. Before his therapist could say anything, the patient announced, "Big deal! There are many fish in the ocean. Girls are a dime a dozen!"

Ongoing comparison between oneself and someone else fueled by envy. The grandiosity manifested by many narcissists is based on a fragile self-concept involving the need to be exceptional and better than others. The maintenance of this structure requires a splitting operation such that others are devalued and seen as "less than" (Stern et al. 2013). Constant comparisons are going on to determine in any interpersonal situation who is "on top" and who is "on bottom." This strategy is doomed to failure as others with admirable qualities begin to threaten the grandiose self of the narcissist, leading to envy, with subsequent devaluation and contempt as a defense against the envy.

Idealization of the other. Kohut (1971, 1977) viewed narcissistically disturbed individuals as developmentally arrested at a stage where they require specific responses from persons in their environment in order to maintain a cohesive self. Those with narcissistic struggles may overvalue others and attempt to create a mutual admiration society. They also may derive enhanced self-esteem by positioning themselves in the shadow of an idealized object who then confers a sense of specialness on them. Fans who follow rock stars or other celebrities may seek to achieve this form of enhanced self-esteem. However, vulnerable narcissists are frequently dissatisfied because of the difficulty in sustaining idealization of someone who possesses the usual human foibles.

Difficulty grasping or caring about the internal experience of others. Research suggests that persons with the NPD diagnosis have problems perceiving and empathizing with what is going on in someone else's mind (Fossati et al. 2017; Ritter et al. 2011). They may have some capacity for cognitive empathy, but emotional empathy is lacking. More to the point, they may simply not care what the other person is feeling. Someone in a relationship or even a casual conversation with a narcissistic individual may feel he or she does not matter. This inability to connect with others may contribute to the isolation of the narcissistic person.

Intrusiveness as characterized by exhibitionistic displays that encroach on others. In an 18-week psychiatric day treatment program, intrusiveness was the interpersonal domain that was most resistant to any treatment offered for patients with narcissistic disturbances (Ogrodniczuk et al. 2009). This feature is related to obliviousness as well because the narcissist's inattention to the needs of others may lead him to focus only on what is important to him. In this regard, such patients are constantly changing the subject back to themselves or telling long-winded stories that put them at the center of the action.

A retreat from social interactions to avoid being vulnerable to humiliation. The hypervigilant or vulnerable narcissist hopes to avoid a narcissistic injury or a humiliating insult by being quiet and retreating into the background in a situation with others. Although this behavior is associated with avoidant personality features, narcissistic persons fear the lack of admiration, whereas avoidant individuals fear lack of acceptance (Ogrodniczuk and Kealy 2013). In therapy, the hypervigilant narcissist may be relatively quiet but is constantly scanning the therapist's nonverbal communications and comments to identify slights or insensitivity.

A feeling of being a martyred victim of mistreatment by others. As noted in Chapter 1, Cooper (1993) identified a variant of narcissistic pathology that is linked with masochism or self-defeating tendencies. Some vulnerable or hypervigilant narcissists position themselves so that they find themselves repeatedly persecuted, insulted, misunderstood, and taken advantage of by others. They repeatedly feel hurt that others do not recognize the extraordinary extent of their suffering and acknowledge their specialness as a result of that suffering.

Initial charm followed by loss of interest in the other. In the first meeting with a high-functioning narcissist, the other person may be charmed and intrigued by how the narcissist listens, talks, and behaves. Many of the smooth narcissistically organized individuals have mastered the art of engaging a person at the first meeting. However, this initial charm gives way to disinterest over time as the narcissist decides that the other person is no longer of any use to him or her. The other person may feel crestfallen, duped, and abruptly dropped.

Deceptiveness and dishonesty coupled with an effort to seduce or cajole the other. At the lower end of the narcissistic continuum, one finds narcissists who have antisocial features and who actively engage with others through deception. They lie and exaggerate the truth in the service of winning over others to their way of thinking or garnering praise and admiration. This mode of relatedness may involve seduction and exploitation without regard to the impact of their behavior on others.

These modes of relatedness do not comprise the entirety of narcissistic interpersonal relations. However, they are prominent themes that emerge when one attempts to treat narcissistically organized patients. These themes are highlighted throughout this volume, although we acknowledge that not all patients' modes of relatedness are covered by these common patterns.

Some of these same themes are contained in the Alternative DSM-5 Model for Personality Disorders in Section III of DSM-5 (American Psychiatric Association 2013). This model delineates two elements of personality functioning: *self* and *interpersonal*. Self is further subdivided into *identity* issues and *self-direction* issues. Interpersonal is subdivided into *empathy* and *intimacy* (see Table 3–1).

DEVELOPMENTAL ROOTS

These modes of relatedness evoke curiosity about their origins in development. Research is in its infancy on the subject of pathological narcissism. Nevertheless, the contributions of experienced clinicians have been valuable to psychotherapists and psychoanalysts who are struggling with what to say or not to say. As noted in Chapter 1, Kernberg (1970) inferred that primary aggression is central to the development of narcissistic organization within the personality. He noted that the aggression could be caused by either constitutional or environmental factors but clearly felt that the derivatives of that aggression, the chronic intense envy and the feelings of inferiority leading to the need to devalue others, arise from within rather than as a result of the failures of parents or caregivers. He suggested that there is a defensive develop-

---

Table 3–1. Elements of personality functioning

Self:

1. *Identity:* Experience of oneself as unique, with clear boundaries between self and others; stability of self-esteem and accuracy of self-appraisal; capacity for, and ability to regulate, a range of emotional experience.

2. *Self-direction:* Pursuit of coherent and meaningful short-term and life goals; utilization of constructive and prosocial internal standards of behavior; ability to self-reflect productively.

Interpersonal:

1. *Empathy:* Comprehension and appreciation of others' experiences and motivations; tolerance of differing perspectives; understanding the effects of one's own behavior on others.

2. *Intimacy:* Depth and duration of connection with others; desire and capacity for closeness; mutuality of regard reflected in interpersonal behavior.

Source. Reprinted from American Psychiatric Association: *Diagnostic and Statistical Manual of Mental Disorders*, 5th Edition, Arlington, VA, American Psychiatric Association, 2013. Copyright © 2013 American Psychiatric Association. Used with permission.

ment of a pathological grandiose self that functions in concert with a tendency to project the devalued unacceptable elements of the self onto others.

Kohut (1971, 1977), by contrast, believed that narcissistic disturbances originate because of the failures of parents or other caregivers to respond to the child's age-appropriate displays of exhibitionism with empathy and love. Moreover, these parents also fail to provide the child with models worthy of idealization. Whereas Kernberg emphasized internal constitutional aggression, Kohut postulated that failures of external figures are primarily responsible for the development of narcissistic disturbances.

More recently, attachment theory has also been used to understand the origins of these characteristic patterns of relatedness. The central tenet of attachment theory is that secure attachment strongly influences the development of internal working models of relationships that are stored as mental schemas and leads to expectations of the behavior of others toward the self. The early work of John Bowlby (1969, 1973, 1980) emphasized that attachment is a biologically based bond between the child and the caregiver that is designed to ensure the safety and survival of the child. Peter Fonagy (2001), an articulate interpreter of the interface between attachment theory and psychoanalytic thinking, noted that in contrast to object relations theory, attachment theory postulates that the goal of the child is not to seek an object but rather to seek a physical state through proximity to the mother/object.

In contrast to object relations theory, attachment theory has undergone rigorous testing in the laboratory. The seminal research by Ainsworth et al. (1978) created an attachment classification based on responses to the *strange situation*. This situation involved toddlers who were separated from their caregiver or mother, which was noted to elicit one of four behavioral strategies. *Secure* infants sought proximity with the caregiver on her return and then felt comforted and returned to play. *Avoidant* behavior was seen in infants who seemed less anxious during the separation and snubbed the caregiver on return. These infants showed no preference for the mother or caregiver over a stranger. In the third category, termed *anxious-ambivalent* or resistant, infants showed great distress at separation and manifested angry, intense, and clingy behavior when the caregiver returned. The fourth group, termed *disorganized-disoriented*, had no coherent strategy whatsoever to deal with the experience of separation.

These four responses to the strange situation have some degree of continuity into adulthood, and these categories of attachment style can be measured with highly sophisticated interviews (George et al. 1996). The four adult categories correspond respectively to the four responses to the strange situation as follows: 1) secure/autonomous individuals who value attachment relationships; 2) insecure/dismissing (or avoidant) individuals who deny, denigrate, devalue, or idealize past or recurrent attachment; 3) preoccupied (anxiously attached) individuals who are confused or overwhelmed by both past and current relationships; and 4) unresolved or disorganized individuals who often have suffered neglect or trauma. It is important to stress that stability of the attachment classification from childhood to adulthood is not absolute (George and Solomon 2008). Events such as parental death, social support, divorce, serious illness in parents or children, and family system disturbances may modify the early attachment pattern, so there is not necessarily a one-to-one correlation.

Fonagy (2001) stressed that there is a substantial research base demonstrating that the attachment status of the parents not only predicts whether a child will be securely attached but also the precise attachment category in the strange situation. Moreover, the attachment strategies appear to be largely independent of genetic influence. Nevertheless, it is also true that biological temperament must be taken into account to some degree because it may influence a child's response to caregiving by an attachment figure (Allen 2013). On the other hand, temperament can be influenced by environmental factors and can change over time because of high-quality caretaking and attachment.

Fonagy and Target (2003) emphasized a linkage between attachment and *mentalization,* which refers to the capacity to understand that one's own and others' thinking is representational in nature and that one's own and others' behavior is motivated by internal states, such as thoughts and feelings (Fonagy 1998). Secure attachment predicts the capacity to mentalize. Caregivers or parents who have good mentalizing capacity can tune into the infant's subjective mental state, helping the infant to find himself or herself in the caregiver's mind and to internalize the caregiver's representation to form a core psychological self. In this manner, a child's secure attachment to the caregiver engenders the child's capacity to mentalize. Through the interaction with the caregiver, in other words, the child learns that behavior can be best understood by assuming that ideas and feelings determine a person's actions. Hence, mentalizing is often referred to as a *theory of mind.* Neuroimaging studies suggest that the medial prefrontal cortex, the temporal lobes, the cerebellum, and the posterior-superior temporal sulcus may all be involved as components of a mentalization network (Sebanz and Frith 2004). Moreover, it appears that true mentalization is not possible until the child is between the ages of 4 and 6 years.

Reflective function is a measure of mentalizing capacity and is defined as a developmental achievement that permits one "to respond not only to other people's behavior, but to his *conception* of their beliefs, feelings, hopes, pretense, plans, and so on" (Fonagy and Target 1997, p. 679). A thoroughgoing assessment of a patient should include the patient's capacity for mentalizing, which involves two variants: 1) automatic or implicit and 2) controlled or explicit (Bateman and Fonagy 2012). *Implicit mentalizing* happens naturally and without effort in ordinary social discourse. *Explicit mentalizing* occurs when reflection and effort are needed to process what is transpiring between two or more people. Another variant, *hypermentalizing,* has been observed in persons who may overthink in an unnecessarily detailed way and draw conclusions that are inaccurate (Bateman and Fonagy 2012).

ATTACHMENT AND PERSONALITY DISORDERS

Research using concepts of attachment theory suggests that attachment security or the lack of it may predict certain types of personality disorder. Much of the link between attachment patterns and personality disorder has come from studies of borderline personality disorder (BPD).

From the Collaborative Longitudinal Personality Disorder Study (Battle et al. 2004), a clear linkage was made between childhood maltreatment and the development of BPD in 600 adults with personality disorder. Given that experiences of abuse and neglect are usually connected with problematic attachment patterns, Bateman and Fonagy (2004a, 2004b) developed a mentalization-based model derived from attachment theory for the treatment of BPD.

Borderline patients have a great deal of difficulty appreciating and recognizing perceived states of the self and others as fallible and subjective. In other words, they struggle to recognize that their representations of reality reflect only one of the range of possible perspectives. Without secure attachment, children have difficulty discerning their own mental states or those of others. Research on BPD patients has linked the categories of preoccupied or unresolved/disorganized to insecure attachment (Alexander et al. 1998; Allen 2001). The failure to resolve trauma appears to distinguish the BPD group from other personality disorders. Early childhood trauma leads to a defensive withdrawal from the mental world on the part of the victim. Hence, many patients with BPD who have been severely traumatized deal with the abuse by avoiding reflection on the content of the caregiver's mind, which prohibits resolution of abusive experiences (Fonagy 2001).

Research on NPD and attachment theory has been more limited. Using data from two randomized controlled trials, Diamond et al. (2014) compared 22 patients with both BPD and NPD with 129 BPD patients without NPD. Compared with the pure BPD group, those patients with both NPD and BPD were more likely to be categorized as either dismissing (avoidant) or "cannot classify." The pure BPD patients were more likely to be classified as either preoccupied (anxiously attached) or unresolved for loss and abuse. However, both sets of patients were found to have a low capacity to mentalize—that is, poor reflective functioning.

Dickinson and Pincus (2003) studied the link between narcissism and attachment styles in a nonclinical population of 2,532 undergraduate students. The investigators used the Narcissistic Personality Inventory (NPI) and the Personality Disorder Interview–IV (Widiger et al. 1995) to conduct interviews of those participants whose scores suggested narcissistic issues. They also used the adult attachment questionnaire (Bartholomew and Horowitz 1991), which proposes a model of four prototypic adult attachment styles: fearful, preoccupied, secure, and dismissive.

When the investigators divided the participants according to whether they were more in line with the grandiose subtype or the vulnerable subtype of narcissistic individuals, they found the following results: the majority of the grandiose group selected secure (60%) or dismissive (16%)

attachment styles rather than fearful (13%) or preoccupied (10%) attachment styles (Bartholomew and Horowitz 1991). On the other hand, as one might expect, the majority of the vulnerable group selected fearful (50%) or preoccupied (13%) attachment styles rather than secure (27%) or dismissive (10%). In the control group, the attachment styles were as follows: secure 53%, fearful 23%, preoccupied 17%, and dismissive 7%. The authors recognized that they were not selecting the subjects according to personality disorder criteria but rather personality styles that reflect grandiose and vulnerable narcissistic traits.

The finding that different subtypes of narcissism may have different characteristic attachment classifications leads directly to the possibility that grandiose or oblivious narcissism may relate to different early family experiences compared with those that predict vulnerable or hypervigilant narcissism. In fact, a longstanding debate in the profession has been whether to attribute narcissism to excessive overindulgence and admiration from parents or to cold, neglectful parenting (Millon and Davis 1996). Otway and Vignoles (2006) sought to investigate what sort of parenting led to what sort of self-disturbance. One hundred twenty participants enrolled on a college campus agreed to take the NPI as well as the Hypersensitive Narcissism Scale (HSNS; Hendin and Cheek 1997). The NPI is better at delineating grandiose or oblivious narcissism, whereas the HSNS was specifically designed to measure covert or vulnerable narcissism. In addition, the subjects characterized 15 items involving recollections of childhood and perceptions of parental attitudes toward them. Finally, two dimensions of adult attachment—avoidance and anxiety—were measured using the Experiences in Close Relationships Inventory (Brennan et al. 1998).

The authors found that attachment anxiety predicted covert or hypervigilant narcissism, but they were unable to find any other relationships between working models of attachment and forms of narcissism. Of particular interest, however, was the finding that recollections of both parental coldness *and* parental overvaluation contributed positively to predictions of narcissism. Moreover, the notions of helicopter parenting and overindulgence of parents, cited in Chapter 2 as applied to millennial narcissism, also received some degree of validation. Otway and Vignoles (2006) made the following observation:

> The fact that both dimensions of childhood recollections contributed significantly to predictions of overt narcissism may help to explain the paradoxical combination of grandiosity and fragility that is so characteristic of adult narcissists. Seemingly, the future narcissist receives constant praise from his or her caregiver but this is accompanied by implicit messages of coldness and rejection rather than warmth and acceptance, and,

thus, we speculate that the praise—which is also indiscriminate—may come to seem unreal. (p. 113)

Moreover, the findings support the notion that we cannot assume that all praise is inevitably beneficial. This formulation is in keeping with Kernberg's (1998) psychoanalytic perspective, which he described as follows: "Fostering the development of a pathological grandiose self are parents who are cold and rejecting, yet admiring" (p. 41).

One other significant finding in the study by Otway and Vignoles (2006) was that both forms of narcissism appear to share origins in childhood. There was not a simple correspondence, as some might have expected, between parental overvaluation and overt narcissism on the one hand and parental coldness with covert narcissism on the other. Of course, given the vagaries of memory, there is an inherent problem when studies rely on retrospective design based on self-reports.

A more rigorous study (Brummelman et al. 2015) was prospective in design. This investigation involved children in the 7- to 12-year age group, when narcissism begins to manifest itself more clearly. In four 6-month waves, 565 children and their parents provided information related to child narcissism, child self-esteem, parental overvaluation, and parental warmth. Narcissism was predicted by parental overvaluation rather than by lack of parental warmth. The children appeared to internalize the parents' views of themselves as superior or special. Positive self-esteem, on the other hand, was predicted by parental warmth, not by parental overvaluation.

This prospective investigation contains a clinically important point about parenting. Just as narcissistic patients can engage in misrecognition of others in their lives, parents can misrecognize their children. Parental overvaluation, which the Brummelman study identified as a major factor in the pathogenesis of narcissism, can be conceptualized as a form of misrecognition. In other words, the parents are looking at their children but seeing them as who they want them to be, not who they are. Part of what parents must grapple with is their own narcissistic needs for their children to be a reflection of themselves.

Although this prospective study points to an understanding of the pathogenesis of narcissism, the exact constellation of attachment styles is not entirely clear. Investigation of 218 psychiatric day treatment programs patients by Kealy et al. (2015) failed to come up with a clear linkage between pathological narcissism and avoidant attachment. As noted in Chapter 1, "Narcissism and Its Discontents," the narcissistic subtypes are moving targets related to a fluctuating self-esteem that is highly responsive to the way that others respond to the patient. Moreover, Dickinson and Pincus (2003) found an association between secure attachment patterns and grandiose narcissism. Thus, one can postulate that some of these individuals may be the higher-functioning type with somewhat more stable internal object relations.

Kealy et al. (2015) emphasized that the grandiosity found in pathological narcissism is not necessarily associated with dismissive/avoidant attachment because it is essentially defensive in nature. Their study of patients in a day treatment program suggested that "Narcissistic grandiosity is associated with representations of the self as inadequate, fearful, and sensitive to rejection. This suggests that vulnerable self-experience—at least in terms of attachment tendencies—appears to be a salient construct with which to understand narcissistic grandiosity" (p. 402). This viewpoint is supportive of the long-standing psychoanalytic perspective that grandiosity is a defensive structure that is an effort to protect the self from underlying insecurity. Hence, even individuals representative of the grandiose subtype may crumble when criticized or slighted.

Meyer and Pilkonis (2012) reviewed the attachment literature with the intent of finding linkages between NPD and attachment theory. They determined that consistently unresponsive, insensitive, and rejecting parenting may lead to avoidant attachment and thus contribute to the pathogenesis of narcissistic personality. However, when they looked at overt or grandiose narcissism separate from covert or vulnerable narcissism, they found a strong linkage between vulnerable narcissism and anxious attachment on the one hand and a somewhat weaker linkage between grandiose narcissism and dismissing/avoidant attachment on the other. They also suggested that individuals in the high-functioning subtype may be less likely to show any form of insecure attachment. Indeed, they may go through their lives feeling as comfortable as other securely attached individuals despite the presence of exaggerated self-importance and a sense of entitlement.

Slade (2014) stressed that there may be a misplaced emphasis on classification when considering the relevance of attachment theory to clinical considerations: "Attachment classifications reflect dynamic efforts to regulate fear and anxiety, and it is these dynamics rather than the categories themselves that deserve our clinical attention" (p. 259). She recommended that therapists make a concerted effort to understand how an adult patient might have responded to threats to safety and fear as a child and attempt to discern how that strategy is occurring in the present. One should also keep in mind that the classifications are not etched in granite—they are malleable because they are responsive to context and to life events (Holmes and Slade 2018). In terms of the pathogenesis of NPD, Slade suggested that narcissistic defenses can be conceptualized as a response to the threat of not being known and/or of being obliterated within the framework of attachment relationships (A. Slade, personal communication, August 12, 2017). These responses can be seen as defenses against a primitive form of annihilation anxiety and, in attachment terms, a threat to fundamental emotional survival (A. Slade, personal communication, August 12, 2017).

Just as attachment classifications are malleable and influenced by context and life events, so are the various categories we apply to narcissistic difficulties. Current psychoanalytic thinking is that the human mind is characterized by multiple self-states (Bromberg 2009), and we must recognize that individuals with narcissistic conditions can look quite different from day to day and from moment to moment depending on what is going on within their own private worlds and within the contexts that surround them.

MENTALIZATION

The combination of attachment disturbances and difficulty in self-esteem regulation with narcissistically organized individuals leads to problems with mentalizing. The overwhelming need for recognition, validation, and admiration makes it extraordinarily difficult for these individuals to contemplate what is going on in another person's mind. The "noise" in the narcissist's head about impressing, seducing, and charming the other person upstages any possibility of quiet reflection regarding the other person's mind as opposed to his or her own. Those who fit the grandiose subtype of NPD are largely oblivious to what is happening in the other person and may even avoid eye contact so that there is no information that would contradict the hope that the other person is smitten and impressed. The vulnerable or hypervigilant narcissist may be more fixated on the other person's response, but his internal distortions and conviction that he is about to be wounded by the response interfere with a reflective understanding of the other person.

Forms of hypermentalizing are often seen in NPD patients. Hypervigilant patients may overfocus on what might be going on in the therapist's mind, speculating on internal processes that are in reality quite unlikely but nevertheless seem to be worth considering. These musings may have a distinctively paranoid flavor: Is the therapist trying to trick me by not saying anything? Is she trying to make me talk so I'll reveal things I don't want to share? Is he figuring out my vulnerabilities so he can force me to confront them? When the therapist actually says something, the patient may feel that there is hurtful intent and will feel like quitting.

Another variation of hypermentalizing is seen in the patient who offers a lengthy narrative that is disconnected from any emotional content and in fact sounds outlandish. Fonagy et al. (2012) regard this variation as a form of *pseudomentalization.* The patient may be functioning in a pretend mode that antedates full mentalization. To the therapist it may seem like a form of mental masturbation that excludes the therapist entirely.

Levy et al. (2015) noted that in narcissistic individuals, brain regions associated with the ability to empathize show both structural and functional abnormalities. Functional magnetic resonance imaging research showed that compared with healthy control subjects, subjects with NPD have smaller gray matter volumes in the left anterior insula, rostral and medial cingulate cortex, and dorsal lateral and medial prefrontal cortex, all areas that are relevant to the capacity for empathy (Schulze et al. 2013).

The findings of imaging studies that there are neuroanatomical differences in narcissistic personalities compared with control subjects raise questions regarding a genetic contribution to pathological narcissism. Indeed, some research suggests a possible genetic component (Livesley et al. 1998; Luo et al. 2014; Vernon et al. 2008). The findings of this research indicate that trait narcissism has the substantial heritability that other basic traits have. Twin studies, however, suggest that attachment classification is not related to heritability—in fact, shared environment influence accounts for the biggest proportion of the variance (Fearon et al. 2006). Roisman and Fraley (2006) conducted a longitudinal study from early childhood and found that the quality of the infant-caregiver relationship could not be explained by genetic variation and that both unique and shared environmental contributions were significant.

In recent years, research on gene-environment interaction has shifted from the stress-diathesis model to the differential susceptibility model (Leighton et al. 2017). There are clear differences between individuals in susceptibility to environmental influences, with some individuals being far more affected than others by both negative and positive contextual conditions. Hence, in regard to the complicated origins of pathological narcissism, all we can say with any certainty is that multiple factors are probably in play and may vary according to the subtype of NPD. Trait narcissism appears to be inherited to some extent. Attachment models also appear to be relevant. Some data suggest the significance of particular types of parenting. However, we also must keep in mind that parents react to particularly difficult traits in their children, so parent-child difficulties must be regarded as bidirectional. No single cause explains the entire clinical picture. We must avoid the reductionism and mother-blaming associated with the era of "schizophrenogenic mothers" and "refrigerator mothers" (linked to autism), undoubtedly one of the darkest moments in the history of psychiatry.

DEFENSES

Personality disorders require lengthy treatment in order to make significant characterological change (Levy et al. 2015). One of the long-standing observations about NPDs is that persons with NPD fend off the observations and interpretations of the therapist and devalue the therapist's help. Indeed, one of the central paradoxes when working with people who have personality disorders is that the individual comes for help but then fights the therapist every step of the way to avoid being helped. Patients come with an array of defense mechanisms that they deploy to avoid anxiety, despair, humiliation, fragmentation of the self, interpersonal closeness, and a variety of other concerns. When the patient enters treatment, defenses manifest themselves as resistances to the therapeutic efforts of the treating clinician (Gabbard 2017). From an attachment perspective, defenses can be understood as a way of finding a workable path between danger on the one hand and safety on the other (Holmes and Slade 2018).

Research on personality disorders (Clemence et al. 2009; Perry et al. 2013) has suggested that a specific set of defenses is common in NPDs. Among the defenses that are commonly used are projection, devaluation, omnipotence, idealization, rationalization, and splitting. Some of these defenses are also typical of BPD, and Kernberg (1970, 1984, 2014) has long suggested that narcissistic patients may have underlying borderline organization.

These defenses are often used as a way of regulating the patient's self-esteem. The pathological grandiose self of the patient is established as a way of avoiding the excruciating humiliation of being inferior, incompetent, unlovable, and deeply envious. Hence, splitting is required to maintain the grandiose self, and projection is used to disavow the negative features that one is dimly aware of and to place them in others. The splitting of the self results in preserving the grandiose self-structure while viewing the devalued aspects of the self as residing in others. Narcissistic patients tend to be externalizers of responsibility and blame. They also disavow undesirable traits in themselves and see them only in others. Rationalization is another defense used to explain away failures of the patient as actually the failures of others.

The defenses of omnipotence and devaluation can also be viewed as part of this overall splitting process. Narcissistic individuals have a desperate need to convince others of their special qualities, and it is often necessary to devalue others to exalt themselves. Idealization as a defense can also be useful, as Kohut (1971) described, in that the patient may need to be in the reflected glory of the other to feel the kind of self-esteem or self-worth that is necessary in order to function.

What is apparent is that beneath the narcissistic defenses there is grave self-doubt, low self-esteem, and insecurity. Research into personality disorders has identified the construct of masochistic self-regard (Huprich et al. 2016). This construct has been linked to the vulnerable subtype of NPD as well as self-defeating personality disorders and individuals with depressive personalities. These individuals tend to be low in self-esteem, hypersensitive to criticism, and frequently shame prone while also having perfectionistic ideas about themselves that are never fulfilled. They often seek to be perfect so they will not be rejected or criticized by others. One could characterize them as lacking in "healthy narcissism" in the sense that they may forgo self-care and go to extraordinary lengths to please others in order to gain approval. Huprich et al. (2016) suggested that masochistic self-regard is at the very core of narcissistic vulnerability. Indeed, a striking feature of the hypervigilant narcissist is to respond to any form of negative feedback, even neutral feedback, as attacking and highly personalized. Hence, the idealization of others can be used as a defense in the service of currying favor and receiving praise from others in order to deal with one's own malignant self-regard.

Another defensive variation is to use projection of the critical features within and regard them as occurring in someone else who is important to the narcissist. This projective process partially explains the hypervigilant attitude of the vulnerable narcissist, who is riveted to the tone of voice, the choice of words, and the nonverbal communication of a significant other in an attempt to detect criticism or contempt. The tendency of hypervigilant narcissists to over-read these attitudes in others leads them to be wary in any close relationship.

The clinician must keep in mind that the modes of relatedness and the associated defenses are all designed to regulate self-esteem, to ward off critical attacks from within and without, and to enable a form of self-deception that cushions the patient from feeling shame and humiliation. This understanding can help the therapist maintain a sense of compassion for the patient's struggle instead of falling into the same pattern as others who are in the patient's life: contempt, avoidance, and dread.

REFERENCES

Ainsworth MS, Blehar MC, Waters E, et al: Patterns of Attachment: A Psychological Study of the Strange Situation. Hillsdale, NJ, Lawrence Erlbaum, 1978

Alexander PC, Anderson CL, Brand B, et al: Adult attachment and long-term effects in survivors of incest. Child Abuse Negl 22(1):45–61, 1998 9526667

Allen JG: Traumatic Relationships and Serious Mental Disorders. New York, Wiley, 2001

Allen JG: Mentalizing in the Development and Treatment of Attachment Trauma. London, Karnac, 2013

American Psychiatric Association: Diagnostic and Statistical Manual of Mental Disorders, 5th Edition. Arlington, VA, American Psychiatric Association, 2013

Bartholomew K, Horowitz LM: Attachment styles among young adults: a test of a four-category model. J Pers Soc Psychol 61(2):226–244, 1991 1920064

Bateman AW, Fonagy P: Mentalization-based treatment of BPD. J Pers Disord 18(1):36–51, 2004a 15061343

Bateman A, Fonagy P: Psychotherapy for Borderline Personality Disorder: Mentalization-Based Treatment. Oxford, UK, Oxford University Press, 2004b

Bateman A, Fonagy P: Handbook of Mentalizing in Mental Health Practice. Arlington, VA, American Psychiatric Publishing, 2012

Battle CL, Shea MT, Johnson DM, et al: Childhood maltreatment associated with adult personality disorders: findings from the Collaborative Longitudinal Personality Disorders Study. J Pers Disord 18(2):193–211, 2004 15176757

Bowlby J: Attachment and Loss, Vol 1. Attachment. London, Hogarth /Institute of Psycho-Analysis, 1969

Bowlby J: Attachment and Loss, Vol 2. Separation: Anxiety and Anger. London, Hogarth/Institute of Psycho-Analysis, 1973

Bowlby J: Attachment and Loss, Vol 3. Loss, Sadness and Depression. London, Hogarth Press/Institute of Psycho-Analysis, 1980

Brennan KA, Clark CL, Shaver PR: Self-report measurement of adult romantic attachment: an integrative overview, in Attachment Theory and Close Relationships. Edited by Simpson JA, Rholes WS. New York, Guilford, 1998, pp 46–76

Bromberg PM: Truth, human relatedness, and the analytic process: an interpersonal/relational perspective. Int J Psychoanal 90(2):347–361 2009 19382965

Brummelman E, Thomaes S, Nelemans SA, et al: Origins of narcissism in children. Proc Natl Acad Sci USA 112(12):3659–3662, 2015 25775577

Clemence AJ, Perry JC, Plakun EM: Narcissistic and borderline personality disorders in a sample of treatment refractory patients. Psychiatr Ann 39(4):175–184, 2009

Cooper AM: Psychotherapeutic approaches to masochism. J Psychother Pract Res 2(1):51–63, 1993 22700126

Diamond D, Levy KN, Clarkin JF, et al: Attachment and mentalization in female patients with comorbid narcissistic and borderline personality disorder. Personal Disord 5(4)428–433, 2014 25314231

Dickinson KA, Pincus AL: Interpersonal analysis of grandiose and vulnerable narcissism. J Pers Disord 17(3):188–207, 2003 12839099

Fearon RMP, Van Ijzendoorn MH, Fonagy P, et al: In search of shared and non-shared environmental factors in security of attachment: a behavior-genetic study of the association between sensitivity and attachment security. Dev Psychol 42(6):1026–1040, 2006 17087539

Fonagy P: An attachment theory approach to treatment of the difficult patient. Bull Menninger Clin 62(2):147–169, 1998 9604514

Fonagy P: Attachment Theory and Psychoanalysis. New York, Other Press, 2001

Fonagy P, Target M: Attachment and reflective function: their role in self-organization. Dev Psychopathol 9(4):679–700, 1997 9449001

Fonagy P, Target M: Psychoanalytic Theories: Perspectives From Developmental Psychology. London, Whurr, 2003

Fonagy P, Bateman AW, Luyten P: Introduction and overview, in Handbook of Mentalizing in Mental Health Practice. Edited by Bateman AW, Fonagy P. Arlington, VA, American Psychiatric Publishing, 2012, pp 3–42

Fossati A, Somma A, Pincus A, et al: Differentiating community dwellers at risk for pathological narcissism from community dwellers at risk for psychopathy using measures of emotion recognition and subjective emotional activation. J Pers Disord 31(3):325–345, 2017 27322580

Gabbard GO: Two subtypes of narcissistic personality disorder. Bull Menninger Clin 53(6):527–532, 1989 2819295

Gabbard GO: Psychodynamic Psychiatry in Clinical Practice: DSM-5. Arlington, VA, American Psychiatric Publishing, 2014

Gabbard GO: Long-Term Psychodynamic Psychotherapy: A Basic Text, 3rd Edition. Arlington, VA, American Psychiatric Association Publishing, 2017

George C, Solomon J: The caregiving system: behavioral systems approach to parenting, in Handbook of Attachment: Theory, Research and Clinical Applications, 2nd Edition. Edited by Cassidy J, Shaver PR. New York, Guilford, 2008, pp 833–856

George C, Kaplan N, Main M: The Adult Attachment Interview. Berkeley, CA, Department of Psychology, University of California, 1996

Hendin HM, Cheek JM: Assessing hypersensitive narcissism: a reexamination of Murray's Narcissism Scale. J Res Pers 31(4):588–599, 1997

Holmes J, Slade A: Attachment for Therapists: Science and Practice. London, Sage, 2018

Huprich SK, Lengu K, Evich C: Interpersonal problems and their relationship to depression, self-esteem, and malignant self-regard. J Pers Disord 30(6):742–761, 2016 26623538

Kealy D, Ogrodniczuk JS, Joyce AS, et al: Narcissism and relational representations among psychiatric outpatients. J Pers Disord 29(3):393–407, 2015 23398104

Kernberg OF: Factors in the psychoanalytic treatment of narcissistic personalities. J Am Psychoanal Assoc 18(1):51–85, 1970 5451020

Kernberg OF: Severe Personality Disorder: Psychotherapeutic Strategies. New Haven, CT, Yale University Press, 1984

Kernberg OF: Pathological narcissism and narcissistic personality disorder: theoretical background and diagnostic classification, in Disorders of Narcissism: Diagnostic, Clinical, and Empirical Implications. Edited by Ronningstam E. Washington, DC, American Psychiatric Press, 1998, pp 29–51

Kernberg OF: An overview of the treatment of severe narcissistic pathology. Int J Psychoanal 95(5):865–888, 2014 24902768

Kohut H: The Analysis of the Self: A Systematic Approach to the Psychoanalytic Treatment of Narcissistic Personality Disorders. New York, International Universities Press, 1971

Kohut H: The Restoration of the Self. New York, International Universities Press, 1977

Levy KN, Johnson VN, Clouthier TL, et al: An attachment theoretical framework for personality disorders. Can Psychol 56(2):197–207, 2015

Leighton C, Botto A, Silva JR, et al: Vulnerability or sensitivity to the environment? Methodological issues, trends, and recommendations in gene-environment interactions research in human behavior. Front Psychiatry 8:106, 2017 28674505

Livesley WJ, Jang KL, Vernon PA: Phenotypic and genetic structure of traits delineating personality disorder. Arch Gen Psychiatry 55(10):941–948, 1998 9783566

Luo YLL, Cai H, Sedikides C, et al: Distinguishing communal narcissism from agentic narcissism: a behavior genetics analysis on the agency-communion model of narcissism. J Res Pers 49:52–58, 2014

Meyer B, Pilkonis P: Attachment theory and narcissistic personality disorder, in The Handbook of Narcissism and Narcissistic Personality: Theoretical Approaches, Empirical Findings, and Treatments. Edited by Campbell KW, Miller JD. Hoboken, NJ, Wiley, 2012, pp 434–444

Millon T, Davis R: Disorders of Personality: DSM-IV and Beyond, 2nd Edition. New York, Wiley, 1996

Ogrodniczuk JS, Kealy D: Interpersonal problems of narcissistic patients, in Understanding and Treating Pathological Narcissism. Edited by Ogrudniczuk JS. Washington, DC, American Psychological Association, 2013, pp 113–127

Ogrodniczuk JS, Piper WE, Joyce AS, et al: Interpersonal problems associated with narcissism among psychiatric outpatients. J Psychiatr Res 43(9):837–842, 2009 19155020

Otway LJ, Vignoles VL: Narcissism and childhood recollections: a quantitative test of psychoanalytic predictions. Pers Soc Psychol Bull 32(1):104–116, 2006 16317192

Perry JC, Presniak MD, Olson TR: Defense mechanisms in schizotypal, borderline, antisocial, and narcissistic personality disorders. Psychiatry 76(1):32–52, 2013 23458114

Pincus AL, Lukowitsky MR: Pathological narcissism and narcissistic personality disorder. Annu Rev Clin Psychol 6:421–446, 2010 20001728

Ritter K, Dziobek I, Preissler S, et al: Lack of empathy in patients with narcissistic personality disorder. Psychiatry Res 187(1–2):241–247, 2011 21055831

Roisman GI, Fraley RC: The limits of genetic influence: a behavior-genetic analysis of infant-caregiver relationship quality and temperament. Child Dev 77(6):1656–1667, 2006 17107452

Ronningstam E: Narcissistic personality disorder in DSM-V—in support of retaining a significant diagnosis. J Pers Disord 25(2):248–259, 2011 21466253

Russ E, Shedler J, Bradley R, et al: Refining the construct of narcissistic personality disorder: diagnostic criteria and subtypes. Am J Psychiatry 165(11):1473–1481, 2008 18708489

Schulze L, Dziobek I, Vater A, et al: Gray matter abnormalities in patients with narcissistic personality disorder. J Psychiatr Res 47(10):1363–1369, 2013 23777939

Sebanz N, Frith C: Beyond simulation? Neural mechanisms for predicting the actions of others. Nat Neurosci 7(1):5–6, 2004 14699409

Slade A: Imagining fear: attachment, threat, and psychic experience. Psychoanal Dialogues 24(3):253–266, 2014

Stern VL, Yeomans F, Diamond D, et al: Transference-focused psychotherapy for narcissistic personality, in Understanding and Treating Pathological Narcissism. Edited by Ogrudniczuk, JS. Washington, DC, American Psychological Association, 2013, pp 235–252

Vernon VA, Villani VC, Vickers LC, et al: A behavioral genetic investigation of the Dark Triad and the Big 5. Pers Individ Dif 44(2):445–452, 2008

Widiger TA, Mangine S, Corbitt EM, et al: Personality Disorder Interview-IV: A Semistructured Interview for the Assessment of Personality Disorders. Odessa, FL, Psychological Assessment Resources, 1995

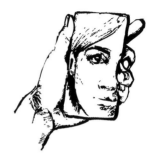

Part II

Treatment Strategies

4

Beginning the Treatment

Dr. A arrives in her office one weekday morning and listens to her voice mail. There are three long messages awaiting her, all from the same person. The first one says, "Hello, Dr. A. I was referred to you by a colleague of yours, Dr. B, who said to say hello to you from him. By the way, he says you are the best. So I have high expectations. I am an extraordinarily busy person, but I have some time available on Fridays at noon, so I would like to see you then. Can we start this Friday? Please call me back." The second message, which is far less formal, begins with his calling Dr. A by her first name: "Hi, Mary. It's Fred again. Just checking to see if you got my message. I was thinking that what I really need from you is a good diagnosis, but I'm not sure if I need treatment. I've seen other doctors, but I think I may have been too much for them to handle." The prospective patient continues to talk, and the message cuts off because of its length. The third voice mail begins with "I forgot to ask you, can you e-mail me your CV? I'd really appreciate it if you would return this call. I haven't heard back from you. Here's my e-mail address."

Dr. A listens to these three voice mails with a deep sense of dread. Part of her wants to avoid returning the call. She questions whether she wants to engage in treatment with someone who has already called three times in 4 hours and is trying to control the treatment from the first phone call. She hears the communications about how others have failed him, and underlying those statements is the implicit question "How can you be different from the previous therapists?" She dreads his going through her curriculum vitae (CV) with a fine-toothed comb, but she realizes that almost anything is available on the Internet these days and assumes she cannot actually hide it from him.

THE FIRST CONTACT

A time-honored clinical axiom is that the way the patient comes to you speaks volumes about who the patient is. That axiom holds up well when the patient who wants to start treatment has narcissistic problems. Patient and therapist both confront a similar situation at the first contact. The patient's difficulty knowing how to relate to others is usually apparent from the beginning. Similarly, from the therapist's perspective, he or she is reacting the same way everyone else reacts to the narcissistic patient. The prospective patient is clearly thinking, "What do I have to do to impress this therapist? Is she going to be good enough for me?" Dr. A is already dreading the first appointment and experiencing the patient's sense of entitlement when she receives three phone messages in 4 hours. She is wondering, "Is this person trying to impress me that he already knows everything there is to know about his illness? Is he trying to take control of this conversation?" The problems that the narcissist encounters in every relationship are thrust on the therapist at the outset, and the therapist is likely to be discombobulated like everyone else is with this person. In short, it's awkward.

The patient wants a copy of Dr. A's CV. It is often of extreme importance for narcissists to see the best therapist in town (even though the idea that there *is* a "best therapist" is nonsense). As Kohut (1971, 1977) pointed out, the patient may want to be in the shadow of an idealized object because that will enhance his self-esteem. The late James Masterson (personal communication, 1988) was once quoted in *The New York Times* in an article about narcissistic personality disorder (NPD). After the article appeared, he received 12 phone calls from individuals who said they read the article and felt that his descriptions sounded like them. Each of them asked if he could treat them. Masterson dutifully returned each call, and in each case his initial impression was that the patients were probably correct that the NPD diagnosis fit them. He told each patient that his practice was full, but he gave them the name of a colleague who was extremely experienced in the treatment of NPD and recommended they call him to start treatment. Out of curiosity, he called his colleague a week later and learned that not a single person had followed up on his referral. If they could not have the "number one expert," they were not willing to try with a lesser being.

WHAT BRINGS A NARCISSISTIC PATIENT TO TREATMENT?

Despite a sense of self-importance, a belief that he or she is special, and a sense of entitlement, it still is not easy for the narcissistic person to deal with his or her failures, losses, and disappointments. Narcissistic injuries that occur in the common, daily disappointments of life can become additive over time and lead the patient to seek out comfort, support, and resolution in psychotherapy. Certainly, major failures and critical life stressors often compel people to seek treatment. The jilted lover, the divorced husband, the person who has just lost her job, the rejected parent, these are all people who may seek out treatment. Table 4–1 offers some profiles of how and why narcissistic patients may come to treatment.

One poignant example is Ms. C, who grudgingly comes to treatment with Dr. D:

> Ms. C enters the room, sets her huge purse down on the floor, and sits on the edge of the couch. She has felt angry, depressed, and empty since her husband left her 8 years ago. "I doubt you can help me. No one can. You probably won't even want to be with me. But I just can't get my mind around it; how could he have left me? I've played it over and over again in my mind. I never should have trusted him, and now I've lost everything." She opens up her purse and takes out a stack of letters and photos. "I carry these in my purse all the time." They are wedding photos, photos of their child, and letters. Love letters from the beginning of the relationship, birthday cards, the letter he left on the kitchen table when he left her, kindly but firmly saying that "I have tried and tried, but you always have to be the victim. No matter what I say, I'm wrong." In the stack is the copy of the divorce agreement and e-mails from her brother saying he wouldn't be there for Christmas and her daughter saying she planned to spend the summer with her ex-husband. The patient lays them all out on

Table 4–1. Patients with narcissistic personality disorder in treatment

Reasons for seeking treatment	Problems, complaints, and symptoms	Personal functioning and life circumstances
Ultimatum or requirements from family, employers, or courts	Denial or lack of awareness of own problems or suffering Unassuming naivete Projection onto or blame of problems on others	Consistent self-enhancing or narcissistically sustained functioning Fluctuations in vocational/professional performance or in collaborative or interpersonal/intimate functioning
Dissatisfaction with life; inability to reach or pursue goals or aspired accomplishments	Absence of major external problems Inner emptiness, meaninglessness, and/or dysphoria Social isolation and inability to form or maintain close relationships Facing limitations or inability to reach goals in personal or professional life	Consistent or high functioning Self-regulatory sustaining interpersonal and/or vocational ability, with areas of success or recognition Internal doubts, self-criticism, distancing, detachment
Acute crises; vocational, financial, or personal failures or losses	Rage outbursts, sexual dysfunction, situational anxiety, insecurity, inferiority, shame, fear	Sudden or gradually developing corrosive life circumstances
Major mental disorder: acute or gradual onset of bipolar disorder, substance abuse, posttraumatic stress disorder, or major depression	Depression, anxiety, rage, or mood lability Growing dependency on alcohol or drugs Sudden memory flashbacks or intrusive thoughts	Self-enhancing function of mood elevation or substance use Reoccurrence of narcissistic trauma Sudden or gradual functional decline

Table 4–1. Patients with narcissistic personality disorder in treatment *(continued)*

Reasons for seeking treatment	Problems, complaints, and symptoms	Personal functioning and life circumstances
Suicidality; acute serious suicidal preoccupation; having survived a lethally intended suicidal effort	Internal despair, fear, overwhelming shame and humiliation, worthlessness, rage	Job loss, financial crises, failed promotion, divorce, loss of significant sustaining attachment or self-regulatory support Other subjectively traumatic or severely humiliating experiences

Source. Reprinted from Ronningstam EF: "Narcissistic Personality Disorder," in *Gabbard's Treatments of Psychiatric Disorders*, 5th Edition. Edited by Gabbard GO. Washington, DC, American Psychiatric Publishing, 2014, pp. 1073–1086. Copyright © American Psychiatric Publishing. Used with permission.

the therapist's couch next to her, the archive of her anger, disappointment, failures, and losses, all carried every day in her handbag.

Many vulnerable narcissistic patients can be grievance collectors
who fit Cooper's (1993) model of the narcissistic-masochistic patient
mentioned in Chapter 1, "Narcissism and Its Discontents." Ms. C's
handbag weighs her down in the same way that her intrapsychic list of
slights, wounds, and mistreatments does. The contents remind her of all
the ways she has lost and all the times people have hurt her feelings. Her
heartaches, disappointments, and narcissistic injuries are all contained
in her metaphoric albatross on her arm. In other patients, grievances are
collected not in a physical way but as emotional baggage or lists presented to others about how they should change. Such patients may list
for the therapist all of the ways that others have failed them. They may
describe arguments with their spouse in which they end up berating
him or her for everything the spouse has ever done to disappoint them
in the context of their marriage. Partners and spouses can feel blind-
sided when an argument about a current event turns into a barrage of
historical slights and disappointments thought to be long forgotten in
the archives of the past. Similarly, in treatment, a therapist who disap-
points the patient may find himself or herself on the receiving end of a
litany of past ways that the therapist has failed the patient.

Some patients come to treatment to deal with a sense of victimization. They feel that the good things in life—jobs, relationships, success,
or even luck—always happen to other people. From the first session, the
therapist is faced with the challenge of empathizing with someone who
feels mistreated, misunderstood, and victimized, while at the same time
pointing out the patient's tendency to externalize responsibility and
shift blame onto others. With this kind of hypervigilant patient, the therapist is aware that the patient is watching his every move. She is tuning
into the therapist with the assumption that it is only a matter of time until
he, too, will victimize her like everyone else in her life does. The patient
wants to know that she is important to the therapist, that he empathizes
with her, and that he is attuned to her feelings. The therapist knows that
this patient will inevitably be disappointed, feel misunderstood, and
even become enraged at him when he makes a misstep (Gabbard 2014).

Some patients experience a feeling of specialness at being mistreated
persistently while holding on to a sense of altruism in their actions (Cooper
1993). These patients may present for therapy ostensibly to change the
family system or their work situation, all in the service of putting a stop
to the victimization. However, they may actually receive a great deal of
personal satisfaction and a feeling of specialness from playing the role

of aggrieved martyr. They desperately need the therapist's validation of their distinction as one who has suffered in a way that is unique and excessive. The internal world of these patients and their motivations will be discussed further in Chapter 5, "Transference and Countertransference."

Patients with narcissistic personality traits often present for treatment of what they view as other conditions. They may be entirely correct. Substance abuse, mood disorders, and anxiety disorders are highly comorbid with NPD (Stinson et al. 2008), and often it is one of these accompanying conditions that prompts the patient to seek help. A sense of failure, narcissistic injury, disappointment, and emptiness may precipitate the symptoms of major depression. There is good reason to believe that narcissistic injuries can also trigger suicide attempts (Links 2013). Narcissistic traits can coexist with bipolar disorder in a way that can make it difficult to tease out the grandiosity associated with a hypomanic episode from the baseline grandiosity inherent in the personality. Anxiety can certainly be heightened in patients with hypervigilant narcissism, as they obsessively tune in to see how others react to them, all the time worrying about criticism and judgment. Alcohol and drug use or sexual promiscuity can fill a void or mute a feeling of failure in someone who is narcissistically organized.

> Mr. D is a 32-year-old man referred for psychotherapy for "sex addiction" at a trainee clinic in an academic medical center. He requested a female therapist. In his first session, he told his therapist that he had sex addiction because he believes he was sexually molested as a small boy. He explained to his new therapist that he had recently completed a month during which he went to bars each evening after work with the intent of having sex with a different woman every night. He said with a broad smile meant to enchant his therapist, "I really love women, and they can see that when they go to bed with me." He has never been married because "not a single woman has measured up to my expectations." The trainee therapist treating him soon recognized that he had a narcissistic personality with utter contempt for women and that he used women and discarded them without the slightest sense of remorse or regret. Mr. D was in a 12-step program for sex addicts, but he attended the group only intermittently because he found that he was not like the other people there, who were all "losers."

At times, the patient who is narcissistic comes to clinical attention in the context of significant family conflict or losses. Certainly, in the process of separation or divorce, the trauma within the family can drive both individuals into treatment, as well as the larger family into therapy. Narcissistic defenses cannot always hold up in the face of painful and significant losses, such as the death of a child or spouse. The narcissistically organized patient may for the first time be feeling pain in a way that he or she cannot manage with his or her usual strategies of denial, avoidance, or projection.

Patients who struggle with narcissistic issues may also have a difficult awakening to the acceptance of limits when they enter middle age.

> Mr. E came to see a therapist for the first time shortly after he turned 50. He spoke with intensity and periodically teared up. He explained that he had been successful in his law firm and loved his family, but he had a nagging sense of dissatisfaction. He lowered his eyes for a moment and then looked up at his therapist, Dr. F. "I fear obscurity," he said. He elaborated by saying, "I'll pass through life like millions of others do, and no one will really know who I am. I feel I haven't accomplished what I thought I would. I wanted to be standing next to a trophy shelf by this point in my life. I need accolades for some reason. I've just come to realize how prevalent my desire to be universally liked and admired is, compared to most people I know. I'm ashamed to say it, but I really wanted to be well known, and I'm not." Dr. F wondered if Mr. E were seeking therapy because he wanted to be "known" in depth by someone. Mr. E thought for a moment and said, "Yes, I would like that. I just don't know what my place is in the universe. I'm haunted by that famous quotation from Joseph Campbell that one should follow his bliss. I haven't been able to do that for some reason. I feel lost." Dr. F asked him what his goals were for therapy. Mr. E reflected a moment and said, "I'd really like to be okay with who I am as I am, but I don't feel I can settle for that. All my life's energy has been associated with a need to prove myself worthy and acceptable. And this could only be measured by how other people react to me."
>
> Dr. F was moved by the poignant way that Mr. E had come to therapy. He felt there was something universal in the patient's striving and in his disillusionment. To some extent, he felt that they were kindred spirits searching for some form of validation and meaning in a complicated universe of unknowns. The wounded narcissism had an appeal to Dr. F that made him eager to embark on the therapeutic journey with Mr. E. Dr. F realized that Mr. E was tormented by the tyranny of an imaginary audience that was a product of his own mind.

The case of Mr. E is particularly meaningful in light of the fact that narcissistic patients often evoke feelings of contempt, boredom, irritation, and dread in therapists. As noted in Chapter 1, they are easily relegated to the *other*, that is, "someone not like me." However, the suffering of the reflective narcissistic patient who feels like a failure may evoke compassion in the therapist. Those who choose to be psychoanalysts or psychotherapists have their own narcissism. They go to work each day with a conscious or unconscious hope that they will somehow rescue others from despair and in so doing lift themselves out of their own existential suffering.

THE PATIENT WHO IS SENT FOR TREATMENT

Narcissistic patients do not always begin treatment of their own volition. It is common for someone with narcissistic issues to be mandated to attend therapy by a spouse or partner, a boss, or a licensing board. Many a referral has begun with a phone call from the patient's spouse or partner, such as in this example:

> My therapist told me to call you. He thought you might be able to help me with my husband. We've been together now for 3 years, and what started off as a wonderful relationship has turned into the feeling that I'm alone in this marriage. It seems like I can't do anything right, nothing pleases him, and I'm starting to realize that it's not all my fault. Although he can be the life of the party and loves to socialize, I feel I'm constantly walking on eggshells waiting for his explosions when I don't attend to his needs.

Although such a phone call from the patient's wife can certainly be seen as an opportunity, it is also a challenge for the therapist and patient who are beginning a journey together. How motivated is the patient? How likely is he to sustain interest in treatment? Will he be able to look at himself and consider his role in the marriage or in his family, or will he solely externalize responsibility for his own actions by blaming others? Sometimes, the phone call comes from the narcissistic individual himself, who begins with, "My wife says I need treatment or she is going to leave. So can I get in to see you tomorrow? I think you'll see that she is the one with the problem."

It is a daunting process to begin treatment with a patient who does not wish to be there. The dance of psychotherapy relies on two willing participants and can come to a halt if the patient does not really want to work. One way to address such a situation is to confront the patient with his ambivalence right from the outset. "I know your wife made the initial call, so how do you feel about being here?" It may also be useful to say in the first meeting, "In my experience, therapy isn't likely to help if you are showing up to please your spouse." The therapist must also keep in mind, however, that resistance to treatment is present in one way or another in every patient who crosses the threshold of the office. Some "involuntary" patients may find therapy useful after discovering that they have a place where the therapist listens to them and tries her best to understand what is going on inside them.

Narcissistic patients also come to treatment at the behest of their employers or external organizations. Physicians who have gotten into trouble due to narcissistic rages characterized by exploding in the hospital and screaming at the staff, as well as those who demean coworkers, may be referred by physician health programs or licensing boards for treatment. Clergy may be told by their congregations that they talk too much about themselves at the expense of addressing needs in the faith community (Crisp-Han et al. 2011). Employers in business or nonprofit settings may refer for "anger management" cantankerous employees who are behaving as if the rules do not apply to them and who throw temper tantrums when they do not get their way.

One dilemma in working with these patients in the therapeutic context is the problem of confidentiality. Although it is understandable to think that the employer would need to know how the patient is doing and if he or she is participating in the treatment, the very idea that the content of that treatment would be reported to an external body is anathema to a confidential treatment. Psychotherapy is less likely to be effective if confidentiality is not preserved. How can a patient with a vulnerable sense of self-esteem realistically address her issues of entitlement and grandiosity, thereby making herself more vulnerable, while feeling that her words could possibly be reported to her employer or a licensing board? In the absence of confidentiality, "as if" therapy may be going on—an artificial and highly filtered variant of true therapy. In the consulting room, the major challenge is accessing the patient's own motivation to look at herself and change rather than simply going through the motions or checking the boxes in order to superficially please the employer (while intending to avoid personal investment in a deeper way). One way to manage a situation in which an external body or employer is involved is to report only whether or not the patient attended the session. No content is reported, nor is there reporting of the progress in therapy.

SETTING THE FRAME

As illustrated in the opening part of the chapter, those patients with oblivious narcissism often come to treatment with a fair bit of entitlement. They may expect their phone calls to be returned immediately. They may demand appointment times that best suit their schedule without taking into account the schedule of the therapist, leaving the disgruntled therapist to think, "Does this guy think he's my only patient?" These patients might have a grandiose expectation about the financial arrangements and treatment, such as expecting not to pay for last-minute cancellations. The pressure on the therapist to be available "whenever I need you" can lead to a feeling in the therapist of being "the help," that is, not a treater but a personal assistant or employee who is available at the whim of the patient, without having any true needs of his own.

In managing the entitlement of narcissistic patients at the beginning of treatment, therapists must be attuned to the subtle and overt pressures being placed on them by the patient. It is essential to clearly set the frame from the outset, explaining and following through with cancellation policies and appointment scheduling that attends to the needs of the therapist as well as those of the patient. Failure to do so can lead to great resentment later in the treatment.

Narcissistic patients can push a therapist to set looser boundaries than is customary for that therapist, or they may cross the boundaries, even from the beginning of treatment (Gabbard 2016). Psychotherapists are vulnerable to submitting to pressures from patients in the service of forming a solid therapeutic alliance or ensuring that the patient will return for the next appointment. In her effort to make a difference and build a therapeutic relationship, the therapist may extend herself beyond her usual therapeutic role and acquiesce to narcissistic demands (Luchner 2013).

One patient requested that the therapist, who was a psychiatrist, prescribe medications that were outside of his usual prescribing practices. Although the psychiatrist did not generally prescribe medications for medical conditions, the patient applied pressure for him to prescribe medications for his hypothyroidism, and the psychiatrist reluctantly complied—only to regret it later. In another case, the therapist felt flattered by the patient's admiration and idealization during the first few sessions. The patient responded positively to virtually every statement made by the therapist and praised him as the "best therapist" in the city. After several sessions, the therapist realized that he had been unconsciously extending the time of the session (Gabbard 2016). Mental health professionals, like everyone else, struggle with their own forms of narcissism.

Inherent in narcissistic forms of psychopathology is the assumption that special arrangements should be made to accommodate the narcissistic patient. Another common demand is for the therapist to agree to see a patient after regular hours because the patient claims that it is impossible to come during the therapist's usual work day.

> In the first session, Mr. G told the therapist that 45 minutes was not long enough to give the therapist sufficient detail about his thoughts. He said he really needed to have a 60-minute session and "would be glad to pay for every extra minute because money is not a problem for me." The therapist was caught off guard and rather impulsively agreed to the arrangement. He regretted it later when Mr. G's exception put him in a po-

sition of having no break between Mr. G's session and his next patient's appointment. He found himself resentful that he had no time to return calls or go to the bathroom.

It must be clarified in the context of this discussion that not all decisions to extend the usual time of the session originate from a patient's narcissistic propensities. At times the therapist may initiate a longer session because it is the best solution for a complex clinical problem. For example, some patients take a much longer period to "warm up" in the session. Others need to include a level of detail that requires additional time.

INITIAL MODES OF RELATING TO THE THERAPIST

As noted in Chapter 3, "Modes of Relatedness," the characteristic modes of relatedness often appear in the first meeting or even in the first phone call. For example, treatment with a narcissistic patient may begin with an interrogation. The therapist may feel scrutinized and judged by such questions as "How old are you? How many people with my problems have you seen? What is your general level of expertise?" Alternatively, the therapist may feel idealized when a patient leads with a testimonial: "I've seen two other therapists, and already I can tell in the first appointment that you understand me better than they ever did." The patient may enjoy basking in the reflected glow of the therapist, viewing herself as enhanced by her proximity to such an extraordinary practitioner. Many, if not all, patients today search for information about their therapist on the Internet long before they come to treatment. The "data" gleaned from online information can be used to criticize or praise the therapist depending on the patient's inclination to compete with or to benefit from the reflected glory of the therapist. In the first session, Mr. G confronted the therapist as follows: "One of the comments about you on the Rate Your Doctor Web site said you looked sleepy in one of the sessions—is that true about you?"

Patients may begin with bragging and name dropping, talking about the very important people they know, their grade point average in college, their prominent friends, or how much money they make. Although boasting can be irritating and off-putting to the therapist, a wise clinician can also quickly begin to see the vulnerable person underneath longing to impress the therapist. Why would one spend time bragging and name dropping unless insecurity lurks beneath the surface?

Some narcissistic patients leave no space for the therapist to speak, ask questions, or engage in an authentic conversation from the outset of therapy. Patients who are oblivious narcissists can perceive it as an irritant if the therapist interrupts their monologues, and they may leave no time or space for the therapist's input. Therapists can feel consigned to a "satellite existence" (Kernberg 1984). The patient may expect the therapist to serve as a silent listener who is not allowed a voice or perspective of his own (Gabbard 2009). Some patients are clear in their wish for a "place to vent" rather than a person with whom to engage in a process of self-reflection and change. The therapist is likely to feel closed out and treated as an object who is allowed to speak only when the patient is finished with his exegesis. One woman began her interactions with the therapist by explaining, "What I don't like about my husband is how he constantly interrupts me. My thought processes are complex and detailed, and if I am interrupted, I cannot find the train of thought again. After I lose it, I feel like I might as well have not spoken in the first place." Patients can feel that they need to rigidly control the session and can tend to go on obsessionally overinclusive diatribes that exclude the therapist from the conversation. When this pattern develops early on in the psychotherapy, it is important for the therapist to find a way to break in and offer his or her perspective on what is going on.

Therapists may respond to the narcissistic patient with unconditional acceptance or with competitive feelings that lead to arguing, both of which can be problematic if taken too far (Luchner 2013). Patients with grandiose narcissism may present with overt competitiveness. At times, that competitiveness can induce a pressure in the therapist to "one-up" the patient to prove his or her own capacities (Gabbard 2009). Such efforts can be a problem early on in the treatment, when the therapeutic alliance may not yet be sufficiently solid to withstand an argumentative confrontation from the therapist.

> Dr. H, a 45-year-old physician, came in for her first appointment with the psychiatrist. She lowered her glasses to the bridge of her nose and looked down her nose with condescension at her therapist. She then began to speak: "I was referred to you because they say I am narcissistic. Fair enough; they can think what they want, but I am dubious. I don't see why it is a problem that I am confident. I am the best at what I do, and I am at the top of my game. I can run a marathon, run the hospital, and run my family. Maybe they are jealous because I just do it better than they do. I've done a lot of reading about psychoanalytic theory. I researched psychoanalysis when they told me I would be seeing you. Do you find your thinking more in line with that of Freud or Jung? Kohut or Kernberg? What did you think of that impressive twin study in 2014 suggesting that narcissism is heritable?" The therapist, feeling vaguely irritated by the patient, felt a wish to compete with the patient, to "one-up" her knowledge and bring her down to size. He had to check his impulse to quote the latest research to her and show off his own theoretical and clinical knowledge.

On the other hand, overempathizing with the patient from the beginning may also set up a problematic imbalance in the treatment. As a therapist recognizes the narcissist's shame and vulnerable self-esteem, there can be too much empathy with the patient's perspective, resulting in collusion with externalization of responsibility in the patient's life. If the therapist always and only empathizes, the patient may not learn to see her own role in the problems in her life.

Several sessions into a new therapeutic process, a therapist began to confront his narcissistic patient, asking her to see the role she played in her marital conflict rather than continuing a litany of complaints about her husband. The patient abruptly looked up at the therapist, saying, "What is the matter with you? You are a therapist! Aren't you supposed to be a cheerleader? I didn't come here for you to tell me I'm doing it wrong."

It behooves a clinician who is beginning a treatment with a narcissistically organized patient to attune himself or herself to the patient's ambivalence about getting "help." Any form of observation, interpretation, or confrontation can be construed by the patient as a blow to the patient's self-esteem. Although these patients may wish for the therapist's input on what is creating problems for them, they are conflicted when they hear that input because it means they are not perfect. In other words, there is another level at which the patient is hoping for admiration and praise rather than insight. He or she may feel deeply hurt by being "pathologized" rather than validated or admired. Therapists need to recognize this tendency and conceptualize the bind it presents for the patient so both parties are aware of it and can collaborate on how to deal with it.

TO TELL OR NOT TO TELL—THE DILEMMA OF DIAGNOSIS

One of the major challenges in working with narcissistic patients is how to respond to the patient who wants to know his diagnosis. It can be daunting to tell someone with a vulnerable sense of self-esteem and hypersensitivity to slights that he has NPD. It can be an equal challenge to deliver the same news to one who is an oblivious, grandiose braggart. Clinicians handle this dilemma in various ways. If one wishes to be candid with a patient, one must keep in mind that narcissism has a pejorative meaning in our culture and is often used as an insult. "He is such a narcissist" is a phrase tossed around in political discussions, in workplace gossip, and in close relationships, usually in an inflammatory and insulting manner. In brief, no one wants to be labeled with NPD.

Ronningstam (2014) points out that integrating the diagnosis of NPD as part of starting the treatment can be challenging. The trait-focused diagnosis can sound terribly critical to a patient who is already anxious and then hears such terms as "grandiose sense of self-importance," "entitlement," and "lack of empathy." What the clinician intends to be informative ends up sounding shaming and insulting. This kind of beginning can seriously impede the formation of a therapeutic alliance.

There was a time in the mental health field when therapists would not use diagnostic terms with their patients. However, the ascendance of the Internet seems to have hastened a change in that practice. Now most patients will want to know, "What's my diagnosis?" Hence, it is important that we as clinicians carefully explain what we mean if we use the term *narcissism*. One strategy is to anchor the patient's struggles with self-esteem in his or her developmental history. By using examples from the patient's own childhood and pointing out past disappointments and narcissistic injuries, the therapist who is explaining a diagnosis of narcissism is starting by empathizing with the patient's life experience. Moreover, it is important to clarify explicitly that when we use the term narcissism, we do not mean it in the insulting way that it is used in the culture but rather as a psychiatric term that refers to a pattern of self-esteem vulnerability, propensity to shame, feelings of entitlement or specialness, and sensitivity to slights and narcissistic injuries. When explaining the diagnosis, the therapist can highlight the patient's particular struggles, often in the patient's own words, so that the patient feels seen, heard, and understood, even in the face of the difficult diagnosis. Finally, an essential part of the formulation should be acknowledgment of the patient's strengths, including areas of high-functioning, altruistic efforts and capacity to help others.

Patients who have more of a pattern of oblivious narcissism or those who have features of aggression, interpersonal exploitiveness, or antisocial tendencies may need to be confronted more directly about personality traits that get them into trouble. It can be helpful to illustrate to the patient how his or her difficulty empathizing with others undermines potentially valuable relationships. Indeed, a productive conversation at the beginning of a treatment can involve an explanation of the concept of mentalizing while pointing out the patient's difficulties in accessing what others are feeling and thinking (Bateman and Fonagy 2012; Fonagy 2001; Fonagy and Target 2003; Gabbard 2014).

Another strategy, particularly useful with hypervigilant or vulnerable narcissism, is to focus on particular problem areas without assigning a diagnosis. For example, one highly vulnerable narcissistic patient opened the door for frank discussion with his therapist by talking about his arrogance. Although the patient had come to treatment for major depression, the therapist was beginning to see the shame, self-criticism, and vulnerability that lay beneath the depression. The patient was clearly hurt that others viewed him as arrogant, which paved the way for a discussion of narcissistic vulnerability. The therapist asked a simple question: "I know you said your friends have called you arrogant. Is this worrying you?" When the patient reluctantly admitted that it was, the therapist went on to acknowledge that everyone has needs for self-esteem and validation and that we often are seeking some kind of response in others by saying things that make us seem arrogant. With some patients who seem particularly prone to shame and humiliation, one can avoid using diagnostic terms and can simply stay at a descriptive level by speaking in "plain English."

As noted in Chapter 1, it is extremely common to see narcissistic patients with an array of obsessive-compulsive and self-defeating traits or histrionic and borderline traits, as well as symptoms of other psychiatric conditions. In such cases, the therapist can focus on the spectrum of personality features rather than focusing exclusively on the narcissistic dimensions of the patient. Clinical experience suggests that many patients can more easily hear the term *narcissistic* if it is accompanied by other traits as well. Both narcissistic and obsessive-compulsive patients are prone to seeking perfection. Hypervigilant narcissists who feel repeatedly slighted may engage in defensive self-defeating behavior to ward off attacks, only to alienate those who might be supportive to them. Experienced clinicians often find that the best approach is a succinct statement such as the following: "Frankly, you don't fit any diagnostic category perfectly." This summary statement can be followed by noting the particular areas of strengths and weaknesses.

THE THERAPEUTIC ALLIANCE

A final and crucial factor in beginning a treatment is to forge a therapeutic alliance with the patient. Research demonstrates that the role of the therapeutic relationship is more important than any specific technique in producing therapeutic outcomes (Butler and Strupp 1986; Horvath 2005; Krupnick et al. 1996; Zuroff and Blatt 2006). Although there are various definitions of the therapeutic alliance, the key components are that the patient feels helped and understood, is attached to the therapist, and has a sense of mutual collaboration in pursuing common goals (Hilsenroth and Cromer 2007).

What a therapist does to build a therapeutic alliance is not mysterious. In fact, there is now a modest body of research that suggests what a clinician can do in the first few sessions to promote the alliance (Hilsen-roth and Cromer 2007). Listening sensitively and conveying trust, warmth, and understanding are central to the process. Another measure to help foster the alliance is to explore the in-session process and the patient's affect in a nonjudgmental manner. Addressing both emotional and cognitive factors is also useful. Finally, therapists can identify new clinical issues in the service of promoting deeper levels of understanding and insight, enhancing the alliance while doing so.

A central feature of the therapeutic alliance is a collaborative pursuit designed to shed light on the patient's motives, conflicts, aspirations, interpersonal patterns, and longings. Unfortunately, many narcissistic patients may present obstacles to that collaborative process because of their fear that they will be made to feel worthless, ignorant, pathetic, incompetent, arrogant, or out of control. NPD patients may also be unwilling or unable to identify their character traits that others see as problematic (Ronningstam 2014). They may actually be clueless about why others react to them the way they do and what they are doing to foster negative reactions in others. They may dismiss complaints about themselves as attacks growing out of envy. They may feel unfairly blamed and "scapegoated." They may threaten to drop out of treatment if confronted too harshly and may have repeated ruptures in any semblance of alliance that is formed (Ronningstam 2014).

A good starting point to build an alliance is to identify specific goals for the treatment, even though the patient may be at a loss to come up with any. By focusing on what causes distress to the patient and to others, gradual progress can be made despite the patient's wish to deny and disavow his or her problems. The patient's inability to see what others complain about may lead to specific work on mentalizing and empathy for others. Dishonesty and deception of the therapist can also undermine alliance building and must be brought out into the open.

Lengthy periods of empathic listening may be necessary to build an alliance when one is working with a narcissistic patient. As Holmes and Slade (2018) noted, "If therapy is to be successful, therapists must first validate the patient's emotional stance, before gently challenging the assumptions that underlie it" (p. 33). Those periods when one serves as a sounding board can be taxing, boring, and seemingly useless. However, clinicians must remember that sitting with the patient and listening is not "doing nothing" (Gabbard 1989). Rather, it involves complex processes that occur regularly as part of psychoanalysis and expressive-supportive psychotherapy. As Poland (2017) has persuasively argued, *witnessing* is a major function of both analytic and psychotherapeutic work. Witnessing includes respectful attention in the context of silent listening where one refrains from making intrusive comments based on one's own perspective. This restraint allows the therapist to grasp the full emotional import of the patient's self-exploration in a mode of engaged nonintrusiveness rather than a version of classical analytic abstinence. The patient knows that the therapist is a separate "other," but it is also clear that someone else is making a concerted effort to understand and contextualize the patient's experience, something that may have been painfully missing in the patient's development. Moreover, the therapist is often serving the crucial function of holding and containing affects that cannot be tolerated by the patient alone.

With narcissistic patients, it is tempting to hear what they say in a judgmental way and view them with irritation, and even contempt, as others do. The therapist can note this temptation and try to keep it under control while recognizing that the patient is someone who is struggling in life and desperately needs help to figure out the "moves" of human relationships and the language of mutuality. To paraphrase Freud, the therapist's task is to pursue a course that is not readily available anywhere else in the "real life" of the patient—a course that seeks to understand, empathize, and collaborate.

REFERENCES

Bateman A, Fonagy P: Handbook of Mentalizing in Mental Health Practice. Arlington, VA, American Psychiatric Publishing, 2012

Butler SF, Strupp HH: Specific and nonspecific factors in psychoatherapy: a problematic paradigm for psychotherapy research. Psychotherapy 23(1):30–40, 1986

Cooper AM: Psychotherapeutic approaches to masochism. J Psychother Pract Res 2(1):51–63, 1993 22700126

Crisp-Han H, Gabbard GO, Martinez M: Professional boundary violations and mentalizing in the clergy. J Pastoral Care Counsel 65(3–4):1–11, 2011 22452146

Fonagy P: Attachment Theory and Psychoanalysis. New York, Other Press, 2001

Fonagy P, Target M: Psychoanalytic Theories: Perspectives from Developmental Psychology. London, Whurr, 2003

Gabbard GO: On 'doing nothing' in the psychoanalytic treatment of the refractory borderline patient. Int J Psychoanal 70(Pt 3):527–534, 1989 2793330

Gabbard GO: Transference and countertransference: developments in the treatment of narcissistic personality disorder. Psychiatr Ann 39(3):129–136, 2009

Gabbard GO: Psychodynamic Psychiatry in Clinical Practice, 5th Edition. Arlington, VA, American Psychiatric Publishing, 2014

Gabbard GO: Boundaries and Boundary Violations in Psychoanalysis, 2nd Edition. Arlington, VA, American Psychiatric Association Publishing, 2016

Hilsenroth MJ, Cromer TD: Clinician interventions related to alliance during the initial interview and psychological assessment. Psychotherapy (Chic) 44(2):205–218, 2007 22122211

Holmes J, Slade A: Attachment for Therapists: Science and Practice. London, Sage, 2018

Horvath AO: The therapeutic relationship: research and theory. An introduction to the special issue. Psychother Res 15(1–2):3–7, 2005

Kernberg OF: Severe Personality Disorder: Psychotherapeutic Strategies. New Haven, CT, Yale University Press, 1984

Kohut H: The Analysis of the Self: A Systematic Approach to the Psychoanalytic Treatment of Narcissistic Personality Disorders. New York, International Universities Press, 1971

Kohut H: The Restoration of the Self. New York, International Universities Press, 1977

Krupnick JL, Sotsky SM, Simmens S, et al: The role of the therapeutic alliance in psychotherapy and pharmacotherapy outcome: findings in the National Institute of Mental Health Treatment of Depression Collaborative Research Program. J Consult Clin Psychol 64(3):532–539, 1996 8698947

Links PS: Pathological narcissism and the risk of suicide, in Understanding and Treating Pathological Narcissism. Edited by Ogrodniczuk JS. Washington DC, American Psychological Association, 2013, pp 167–181

Luchner AF: Maintaining boundaries in the treatment of pathological narcissism, in Understanding and Treating Pathological Narcissism. Edited by Ogrodniczuk JS. Washington DC, American Psychological Association, 2013, pp 219–234

Poland W: Intimacy and Separateness in Psychoanalysis. London, Routledge, 2017

Ronningstam EF: Narcissistic personality disorder, in Gabbard's Treatments of Psychiatric Disorders, 5th Edition. Edited by Gabbard GO. Washington, DC, American Psychiatric Publishing, 2014, pp 1073–1086

Stinson FS, Dawson DA, Goldstein RB, et al: Prevalence, correlates, disability, and comorbidity of DSM-IV narcissistic personality disorder: results from the wave 2 national epidemiologic survey on alcohol and related conditions. J Clin Psychiatry 69(7):1033–1045, 2008 18557663

Zuroff DC, Blatt SJ: The therapeutic relationship in the brief treatment of depression: contributions to clinical improvement and enhanced adaptive capacities. J Consult Clin Psychol 74(1):130–140, 2006 16551150

5

Transference and Countertransference

When narcissistic patients seek treatment, the modes of relatedness discussed in Chapter 3, "Modes of Relatedness," come alive in the consulting room between patient and therapist. In the transference-countertransference matrix, the intrapsychic and interpersonal struggles that these patients face in their lives become evident. The therapist, who may be treated with contempt, dismissiveness, and condescension, feels as if he or she is a "function" rather than a person. Skilled and caring clinicians may lose their empathy, use confrontation in a retaliatory manner, withdraw altogether, or watch the clock in eager anticipation of the end of the hour. In short, the narcissistic patient may bring out the worst in the therapist. This common clinical challenge highlights the struggle for those who venture into a treatment process with a narcissist—how can the therapist work to improve the patient's ability to develop stable and fulfilling relationships when the very mode of interaction is off-putting, infuriating, and distancing to the therapist, as it is to everyone else in the patient's life? A brief clinical illustration will demonstrate how the "bad object" becomes the "bad therapist."

> Ms. I started seeing Dr. J in twice-weekly therapy because of her concern that she was being treated badly in her relationships. She wondered what was wrong with her choices. She told Dr. J that she had done everything possible to attract the right kind of man, but nothing was working. A tear came out of her eye as she explained to him, "I'm funny, I'm smart, I spent thousands on a nose job, and everyone raves about my hair. What am I missing?" Dr. J replied that he didn't know. In fact, it was too early to figure out all the reasons for her choices and why certain types of men were drawn to her. He went on to say that the two of them would have to collaborate on a search for answers to that question and others.
>
> From early in the therapy, Ms. I would scrutinize Dr. J's face for any sign that he might be growing disenchanted with her. In one session she stopped talking abruptly and said, "You're not listening to me. Your eyes glazed over!" Her tone was indignant and accusatory, and Dr. J felt he'd been caught. She was right. He had been elsewhere in his thoughts. He felt cornered and knew that denying the truth of what she observed would only make things worse. So after a pause, he made an attempt to be honest but gentle: "You are right. I was lost in thought for a moment. But I try to listen in a way that allows me freedom of thought—I follow my associations to your comments and see where they lead." Ms. I glowered at him. "Isn't this therapy about *me*? Aren't you supposed to be a good listener?" Dr. J felt pinned down by Ms. I. He was growing increasingly irritable, but he maintained his composure and said, "Good listening in therapy may include taking other thoughts into consideration." Ms. I sulked and said, "Nice try to get out of it. You know what you did."
>
> Dr. J was increasingly perturbed, but he managed to maintain his professional demeanor. He was not successful in his effort to do a rupture and repair scenario. He thought to himself, "No wonder she has problems with men. No one wants to be controlled like this." She stared at him and said angrily, "I just think if I'm paying you the fees you expect, I can expect to have your full attention!" Dr. J responded in an irritated voice: "I understand. You don't need to repeat it!" As soon as the words were out of his mouth, Dr. J knew he had lost it a bit. He felt a sense of shame that he had allowed himself to be provoked in that way. Ms. I looked hurt and said, "Now I feel you're scolding me for calling you out." Dr. J said, "I'm sorry," and Ms. I went on after collecting herself

a bit. The session ended uncomfortably, and Dr. J went on thinking about Ms. I as he was driving home from the office.

As Dr. J reflected on what had happened, he recognized that he had been colonized by Ms. I. Her accusations, which had a kernel of truth in them, induced the same reactions in him that she described in other men. He felt cornered, accused, and humiliated. The "bad" internal object within Ms. I had been projected into him and then had taken him over as she applied interpersonal pressure on Dr. J to "admit" what he'd done. Dr. J was well aware that he had a "hook" based on his own subjectivity that provided a convenient landing place for the projected object. Ms. I had unconsciously created a scenario in which her hypervigilant anxieties were confirmed in the transference-countertransference realm. Her scanning of the therapist's face to look for subtle clues regarding disengagement evoked a response that was exactly what she was looking for. Dr. J realized why one man after another felt like disengaging from her. He particularly regretted his irritable outburst in which he said, "You don't need to repeat it!" The colonization by the "bad object" had led him to become a "bad therapist."

In the treatment of narcissistic patients, there are long periods of time when the therapist or analyst must tolerate and "live with" intolerable feelings projected by the patient. The capacity of the therapist to tolerate such intense feelings may in and of itself be therapeutic for the patient. The patient's observation of his or her therapist's attempts to deal with feelings regarded as intolerable makes those feelings somewhat more tolerable and accessible for reintrojection (Carpy 1989).

This form of containment can be broken down into a set of activities when the therapist may appear to be doing nothing (Gabbard 1989). Therapists can use the countertransference to enhance their understanding of the internal object world of the patient. Therapists can also find an analytic space to engage in a quasi supervisory process that involves an inquiry into what has been touched within them by the patient's projections. In addition, they can formulate possible interpretations before actually saying them. In such situations, it is preferable to engage in silent interpretation a few times before actually verbalizing what one wishes to say to the patient.

Perhaps the central point of the therapist's activity is to recognize that what is transpiring between the two members of the dyad illuminates in vivid detail the major internal object relationships that haunt the patient. In the case of Ms. I, she has re-created the victim narrative that has been with her throughout her life. Those who try to help her or love her always fail her.

This form of hypervigilant narcissism with strongly masochistic features can be understood by using W.R.D. Fairbairn's object relations theory as a conceptual framework. Unlike Melanie Klein, who argued that the "bad" maternal object is projected out, Fairbairn (1944/1952) insisted that the mother who is experienced as incapable of providing the infant with unconditional love is internalized. Fairbairn suggested that the child takes the "unloving" mother within, hoping to be able to control her. The child does not give up the need or wish to transform the "bad" mother into a "good" mother. In fact, one can view the infant's wish to transform unsatisfying objects into loving and satisfying objects as the most powerful motivation to create and sustain a highly structured and repressed internal world.

The central ego of the child represses two sets of internal object relationships. One involves an exciting but ultimately disappointing maternal object in relationship to a vulnerable self, and the other is characterized by a rejecting maternal object in relationship to a rejected self (what Fairbairn called the "internal saboteur"). Indeed, Fairbairn (1944/1952) argued that the splitting is necessary because the essential "badness" of the object is precisely due to the fact that it combines frustration and rejection, on the one hand, with allurement and titillation, on the other. Fairbairn described a pathological form of love in the bonding between the rejecting object and the rejected self (internal saboteur). This bond is based on a thoroughgoing resentment. As Ogden (2010) described it:

> The rejecting object and the internal saboteur are determined to nurse their feelings of having been deeply wronged, cheated, humiliated, betrayed, exploited, treated unfairly, discriminated against, and so on. The mistreatment at the hands of the other is felt to be unforgivable. An apology is forever expected by each, but never offered by either. Nothing is more important to the internal saboteur (the rejected self) than coercing the rejecting object into recognizing the incalculable pain that he or she has caused. (p. 109)

Hence, a patient like Ms. I is highly invested in the masochistic victim role and equally invested in letting Dr. J know how mistreated she feels. She wants to be certain that he knows that he has hurt her deeply by not paying rapt attention to her every word. He has become one more figure who raised hope in her only to ultimately fail her like the others. Those on the receiving end of her accusations may experience her as sadistic as well as masochistic. Cooper (2009) viewed this sadomasochistic configuration as constituting the core of narcissistic-masochistic character. Such patients are searching for a "bad-enough object" (Rosen 2013) that will re-create the "badness" of the internal unloving mother and reproduce the complex pleasures of the martyred victim.

This situation sets up what Jessica Benjamin (2018) refers to as a problem in recognition to which both therapist and patient contribute. Ms. I, for example, feels mistreated and neglected by Dr. J., who, in a complementary manner, is angry and struggling with a wish to retaliate. Benjamin (2018) cautions that the mature view of the other as a "like subject" with an "other mind" is repeatedly at risk of breakdown into a complementarity of "doer and done to." The beleaguered therapist may relegate the patient to the role of an object to be controlled or managed instead of another mind with which one can connect.

The therapist must strive to maintain the recognition between sameness and difference while acknowledging the other to be an equivalent center of initiative (Benjamin 2018). As Dombek (2016) argues, the Narcissus myth itself is really about misrecognition. Narcissus thinks he sees another boy just like him, when it is really only his reflection in the water. One could say that Dr. J and Ms. I have engaged in a moment that involves both misrecognition and recognition. In the case of Ms. I, she accurately notes that Dr. J's thoughts are wandering but views him as callously uninterested in her. Dr. J, on the other hand, sees Ms. I as excessively demanding and controlling but misses the poignance of her need to be heard and understood. Recognition involves being genuinely known and "seen" by the other member of the dyad. There is a sense that intentions are understood and that each matters to the other. Benjamin (2018) persuasively points out that therapists and analysts, because of their need to be "healers,, can feel victimized and thus blame the patient for impasses in which recognition and the therapeutic role are taken away from them.

Because of the fact that none of us can observe ourselves in a completely unbiased manner, a consultant can be of great value in these times when there is a loss of recognition in the dyad. Someone outside the dyad may have clearer vision that enables her to see the analyst's vulnerability and his wish to cling to the "paradise lost" of the idealized state of relatedness that may have preceded the collapse. A consultation may open the space for the therapist to explore the rupture with the patient and engage in what is similar and different about the perceptions of the two parties. Such examination may restore the sense of "like subject" even in the face of ongoing disagreement.

The case of Ms. I is emblematic of a recurrent challenge for the therapist, namely, when one becomes colonized by what the patient is projecting, how quickly can one recognize what is going on and address it with the patient? The answer varies, of course, depending on who the analyst is and the nature of the "dance" that has emerged between the two parties. The analyst has to allow herself to be caught up in the moment and allow herself to be carried away to some extent by the music of the session (Gabbard and Ogden 2009). The analyst's aliveness may depend on her willingness and ability to improvise without being sure where things are going (Ringstrom 2001). We further elaborate on these dilemmas in Chapter 6, "Tailoring the Treatment to the Patient," and Chapter 7, "Specific Treatment Strategies," but here we simply wish to introduce the kinds of enactments produced by the transference-countertransference themes in treatment and identify common variations.

The entanglement of Dr. J and Ms. I captures one example of a transference-countertransference enactment typical of a treatment involving a narcissistic patient. In this chapter we briefly elaborate on others. In Chapters 6 and 7, we discuss strategies for dealing with some of the more difficult situations that are likely to arise from the transference-countertransference developments.

History of Transference-Countertransference With Narcissistic Patients

Freud (1957) first developed the term *countertransference* to refer to the analyst's transference to the patient and conceived of countertransference as an obstacle or impediment to the progress of the treatment. In the narrow view of countertransference, closest to the Freudian perspective, the patient is regarded as someone from the therapist's past, that is, the analyst's transference to the patient.

The contemporary view of countertransference has expanded to encapsulate both the narrow version and the broad view (Gabbard 1998, 2013, 2014), which grew out of the work of Heimann (1950) and Winnicott (1949), who both saw countertransference as an important communication from the patient that reveals to the therapist something about the patient's inner world.

In the contemporary intersubjective discourse, most clinicians appreciate that countertransference is inextricably intertwined with transference and that both are jointly created by the patient and the therapist acting in tandem. The patient's transference to the therapist, shaped by his or her own past relationships, induces a set of feelings in the therapist, which are in turn influenced by the preexisting internal object relations of the therapist.

Projective identification, a concept that has evolved over time, was first developed by Melanie Klein (1975) and then expanded by the British Independents. It crossed the Atlantic when Ogden (1979, 1982) elaborated the clinical understanding in a way that brought it squarely into the discourse of American psychoanalysis. In brief, positive identification is now viewed as a vehicle by which the therapist comes to know the inner world of the patient. Through interpersonal pressure in the here and now of the clinical setting, patients unconsciously attempt to impose on the therapist a particular way of responding and experiencing. In so doing, the patient induces the therapist to re-create patterns of relatedness in the treatment relationship that are present in the patient's daily life and past. Hence, the therapist can begin to feel much the way others do in the patient's life when they interact with him or her. Dr. J, in the earlier vignette, for example, started to feel like one of Ms. I's disgruntled boyfriends.

In the current theoretical milieu, transference and countertransference do not exist independently but rather exist together in a complex intersubjective space in and between the patient and therapist. In that regard, most psychoanalytic clinicians today would agree that there are two "patients" in the room. The dyad of patient and therapist is constantly created and re-created through this process.

Freud's (1963) early thinking about narcissism was based on an economic model of the mind that focused on drive cathexis and mental energies. Within that framework, he concluded that narcissistic patients were not amenable to psychoanalytic approaches because they did not have the capacity to develop the classic features of a transference neurosis (Freud 1963). Brenner (1982) elaborated on Freud's initial view by clarifying that the apparent absence of transference *is* the transference in many narcissistic patients. Freud and Brenner both were reacting to a central feature of many narcissistic patients: an apparent lack of interpersonal connection. A major strain on the therapist's capacity to stay attuned in the treatment is the notable absence of mutuality and reciprocity. Compounding this strain is the difficulty that the narcissist has in using the person of the analyst as a vehicle for change.

In his revision of Freud's ideas in the 1970s, Kohut (1971, 1977) expanded our view of narcissistic patients. The therapeutic action was linked to addressing deficits in the patient's self-esteem and self-cohesion. Kohut noted that the patient attempted to fill these deficits through use of the therapist as an extension of the self. He posited that narcissistic patients did, in fact, develop transferences in the clinical setting. He defined these as *selfobject transferences*, by which he meant that the analyst performs functions that are absent in the patient. Kohut conceptualized three variations: mirror transference, idealizing transference, and twinship transference (Kohut 1971, 1977, 1984). *Mirror transference* describes the patient's attempts to gain the admiration, warmth, and validation from the therapist, a repetition of the childhood search for the gleam in mother's eye. *Idealizing transference* puts the therapist on a pedestal and enables the patient to bask in the reflected glory of the idealized clinician, much as a child idealizes a parent. In *twinship transference,* the patient identifies with the therapist as a twin, someone whose inner world is identical to his or her own. Kohut viewed the tendency for patients to dissolve into tears and/or rage as a response to the analyst's failure to meet their needs for mirroring, admiration, and appreciation. He stressed the need for a treatment that focuses on empathy for the patient and understanding of his or her inner world (Kohut 1971, 1977, 1984; Liberman 2013).

In contrast to Kohut's views, Kernberg (1970, 1974, 1975) approached the understanding of the patient from a theoretical perspective that was rooted in ego psychology and object relations. He delineated the aggressive, envious, and even sadistic narcissist who devalues the clinician and seeks to spoil the interpretive approach of the analyst. Although Kernberg acknowledged transferences that shared the phenomenological features of Kohut's mirroring and idealizing, he saw those features as defensive structures behind which rage, envy, and contempt were concealed (Kernberg 1970, 1974).

Kernberg perceived the disengagement of the narcissistic patient as related to the denigration and devaluing of the therapist. This need to depreciate is based in the patient's envious response to the analyst's ability to offer help and insight, which the patient is unable to do for himself or herself. Moreover, this form of resistance is also related to the pseudo self-sufficiency described in Chapter 3 (Kernberg 2014). To feel dependent on the therapist would be the ultimate feeling of being "less than."

THE HIGH-FUNCTIONING NARCISSIST

As we mentioned in Chapter 1, "Narcissism and Its Discontents," the research of Russ et al. (2008) suggests a third type of narcissist, the higher-functioning variant who leads with an engaging exhibitionism enhanced at times by a charm that masks the patient's narcissistic core. These patients wish for the therapist to enjoy, compliment, and admire them. They like to be the "life of the party" and command the center of attention. They try hard to gain respect and impress others while mentalizing enough to know when they might have gone too far and alienated members of their "audience."

The literature on treatment of narcissistic personality disorders (NPDs) is replete with discussions of the transference and countertransference from the perspectives of Kohut and Kernberg. However, little has been written about these phenomena in the high-functioning variant, the smooth and charming narcissist (Gabbard and Crisp-Han 2016). This third subtype is not simply an attenuated form of the hypervigilant or oblivious narcissist, although some traits of both subtypes may appear over time. The primary interest of the high-functioning narcissist may be a form of conquest or seduction—therefore, the transference comes across as a quest to make the therapist succumb to the patient's charm and thus win the therapist's admiration. Winning over the therapist trumps any concern about understanding oneself or making changes in one's life. This dimension distinguishes the third subtype from what is generally regarded as "healthy narcissism," often seen in highly successful professionals who are at least ambivalently seeking out insight and help with a desire to change.

When the high-functioning narcissist first comes to treatment, the transference to the therapist is one that a clinician would expect to see from a high-functioning *neurotic* patient. He or she appears to respect the therapist's point of view and sees the therapist as someone who can potentially help him or her. The countertransference of the therapist is initially positive—the therapist looks forward to seeing someone who is engaging, self-reflective, motivated, and collaborative in treatment. Over time, this positive transference-countertransference dynamic begins to crumble when the therapist realizes that the patient is highly self-referential, and every story features the patient as the pivotal character in the drama and even something of a hero. The therapist gradually realizes that there is a lack of mutuality that previously went unnoticed.

These patients appear to accept what the therapist says, but they do not return to the next session with some form of narrative continuity that is collaborative with the therapist's perspective. This discontinuity from session to session is a major form of resistance in these patients. The therapist notices that his or her observations, insights, and questions are not brought up from week to week, almost as if the therapist and the past conversation have vanished from the mind of the patient within minutes of leaving the session. From the perspective of the patient, the treatment is not based on providing understanding. Rather, it is an ardent wish to gain special recognition, that is, to be the favorite patient of the therapist. It may appear that the patient's overarching goal is to be seen as someone without significant psychopathology who really needs no treatment at all. This transference is fundamentally different from that of the hypervigilant narcissist, who is trying to avoid being slighted rather than gaining admiration.

Whereas the grandiose narcissist is oblivious to the presence of the therapist, the smooth-talking and high-functioning narcissist is highly attuned to the therapist and can follow social and interpersonal cues with grace. Unlike the grandiose and vulnerable transferences, this form of transference flies under the radar for a significant amount of time because the patient is more interpersonally savvy and has a history of winning others over to his or her point of view. These patients are far less likely to dissolve into tears when their feelings are hurt or become rageful when wounded. Moreover, they do not screen out or ignore the therapist the way the oblivious narcissist does. At least superficially, they appear to hear and acknowledge the therapist. They smile, make good eye contact, compliment the therapist, and seem interested in the therapist's insight, but they do not seem to take it in or build on it.

We conceptualize this variant as an example of the false self described by Winnicott (1965). In his description of a developmental problem in the mother-child dyad, the child feels that he must comply with the mother's distorted image of him and splits off the true self in the service of adapting to the mother's expectations. In other words, the patient unconsciously tries to persuade the therapist that he is not self-absorbed or insensitive to others in the service of masking his narcissism and winning over the therapist's admiration. He will try to win over the therapist in the same way he hoped to win his parent's affection.

The false self presentation is a form of self-deception as well as "other-deception." The effort to win over the therapist is an ingrained, automatic adaptation that is not consciously conniving in the way that an antisocial patient might approach a therapist. These high-functioning people are often highly successful in their careers but have problems with interpersonal relationships despite appearing socially smooth. Early in the development of his psychoanalytic perspective on personality disorders, James Masterson (1981) wrote that both borderline and narcissistic personality disorders seemed to involve false self adaptation to please the parents.

The countertransference with the high-functioning narcissist is one that shifts over time, often from being charmed to feeling chilled. The therapist begins the treatment with high expectations of a collaborative process, feeling entertained and connected. The patient may be "special" in some way to the therapist, and there is a sense of eager anticipation when it is time for the patient's appointment. With this type of patient, however, there is a growing recognition that the patient is not actually interested in the inner worlds of others, unless they are a reflection of the patient. The therapist's countertransference gradually, and reluctantly, shifts to a set of feelings. The therapist may feel a poignant sense of empathy for the patient's struggles to hide his or her emptiness or a sense of feeling duped and misled. The therapist realizes that the patient is wearing a neurotic costume that masks a narcissistic structure underneath. This gradual realization can lead to the therapist's slow disengagement and disillusionment regarding the prospects for the therapy.

> Mrs. K, a woman in her 40s, came to treatment with Dr. L in order to work on her relationships. She had had a falling out with her daughters, who were now not speaking to her, and she wanted to try to repair their relationships and become close again. Dr. L was not certain initially what had caused the problems in the family—in his opinion, Mrs. K seemed to have good insight about her children and by her account had acted reasonably. Still, he wanted to learn more. In the opening weeks of the therapy, Mrs. K approached the therapeutic relationship with a sense of vivaciousness. Despite her worries about her family, she was able to be happy about her successes in management at a large company. She was lively, and Dr. L looked forward to seeing her each week. In their sessions, she was funny and engaging, humble at times, and able to laugh at herself.
>
> Over time, however, he started to realize that she placed herself at the center of all of her stories, even more so than with most of his other patients. Rather than a back-and-forth dialogue in the therapy, Mrs. K tended to regale Dr. L with elaborate (although lively) stories that always centered on herself as either the heroine or the victim of the narrative. Although Dr. L laughed, he also realized at the end of the hour that he tended to be distracted by the stories to the point that he was colluding with Mrs. K's avoidance of looking at the role she played in the conflict with her daughters and others in her life. He noted that she was able to depict others with a sense of clarity, to see them for who they were, but somehow the perspective always reverted to her own. Dr. L still enjoyed his time with Mrs. K and still felt engaged in helping her, but he began to feel more marginalized and less connected to her, much as he imagined others in her life must come to feel over time. It seemed that she was more interested in entertaining him than in truly learning about herself or seeing her own weaknesses or faults.

COMMON PATTERNS OF TRANSFERENCE-COUNTERTRANSFERENCE WITH NARCISSISTIC PATIENTS

In describing various transference-countertransference patterns in working with narcissistic patients, one cannot necessarily predict with any degree of accuracy which variation will appear in any given clinical dyad. Both transference and countertransference are idiosyncratic to some extent in that they are based on the past experiences of both therapist and patient. As noted previously, although some patients may initially appear as oblivious or grandiose and others as hypervigilant or vulnerable, these subtypes are fluid in nature and may shift abruptly depending on context and overreaction to the therapist's interventions. The grandiose shell sometimes cracks to reveal a hypervigilant sense of shame and guardedness underneath. The fragile hypervigilant narcissist can at times erupt in volcanic rage, grandiosity, and contempt. A high-functioning subtype can unravel in the face of a mistake or misattunement on the part of the therapist or as a result of a narcissistic injury outside the therapy.

Although research is limited in this area, Betan et al. (2005) asked 181 psychiatrists and clinical psychologists in North America to complete a battery of instruments on a randomly selected patient under their care as part of a study on personality pathology and countertransference. The hallmarks of countertransference to narcissistic patients in this investigation were feelings of being devalued and criticized by the patient, accompanied by anger, resentment, and dread in working with such patients.

In a more recent examination (Tanzilli et al. 2017), 67 psychiatrists and clinical psychologists completed a set of instruments to assess their patterns of countertransference with patients who had NPD. Narcissistic patients evoked angry/hostile, helpless/inadequate, criticized/devalued, and disengaged countertransferences in the clinicians. Positive responses in the therapists were rare. The countertransference patterns were not strongly influenced by the variables of the therapy or the clinicians, although clinical experience was an exception. Some of the clinicians felt insecure and ineffective as part of their countertransference pattern.

The authors noted that the countertransference phenomena seemed to reflect specific aspects of the patient's attachment patterns. In concordance with some of the attachment studies, narcissistic individuals seemed to demonstrate a dismissing attachment characterized by an inflated representation of the self and a defensive detachment from relationships in which other people are seen as irrelevant.

Although these empirically based patterns of response to narcissistic patients are useful for clinicians to keep in mind, highly individualized reactions are likely to occur as well. Given the unpredictability of what happens between two persons engaged in a psychoanalytic or psychotherapeutic process, the best we can do is describe some of the most common patterns of transference-countertransference.

TREATING THE THERAPIST LIKE A SOUNDING BOARD

At times when the therapist is being talked at rather than talked to, he or she may feel a creeping sense of boredom, disengagement, and even sleepiness. The feeling of a "satellite existence" as coined by Kernberg (1970) can lead to mind wandering on the part of the therapist. She may find herself thinking about the next patients on her schedule, or her mind may wander outside the office to her to-do list for after work or what she plans to have for dinner that evening. She may then feel guilty when she realizes that her mind wandering is moving beyond a useful clinical reverie toward disengagement. Steiner (2006) observed that therapists treating narcissistic patients feel chronically excluded. They may react to this exclusion by forcing themselves back into the dialogue. Alternatively, they may become overly judgmental or assertive, resulting in a clinical blunder. Therapists who are oscillating between bored distance and overly zealous interpretation in order to break into the monologue may speak before fully thinking through the consequences of their comments. The therapist may feel like blaming the patient for his boredom, but of course, the patient has no obligation to entertain the therapist. Moreover, it is the therapist's responsibility to remain alert, engaged, and clinically focused. Rather than just telling herself to pay attention, the therapist can use the countertransference of boredom or distance to learn how others in the patient's life feel when he is droning on and help the patient understand some of the reasons for his failure to elicit the responses he desires in others.

PULLING FOR AN EMPATHIC ADMIRING RESPONSE

Narcissistic patients often have a desperate wish for the therapist to admire them, praise them, empathize with them, and recognize their specialness. They are seeking that maternal affirmation that Kohut described. The therapist may or may not oblige with an admiring countertransference. At the most extreme, this wish for admiration comes across as bragging or desperate neediness. Therapists tend to want to hear about the patient's good news and successes, and they often appreciate and feel proud of the patient, even impressed by his or her accomplishments. Kohut's (1971, 1977) work was founded on the understanding that some degree of empathy is necessary to stimulate further growth of an insufficiently developed self. Over time, however, the therapist can feel irritated by the constant pull for mirroring. She can become drained, feeling that she has a limit to her empathy, only to have the patient ask for more. One patient described the wish for reassurance as a "thirst" and another noted that the need for praise "just feels like a hole that can never be filled" (Kohut 1971).

The pull for empathy may begin to feel like a demand, as if the patient is saying, "I need a specific type of empathy from you in exactly the words I want and with the perfect expression on your face, and if you don't give it to me, I am leaving." As a result, the therapist can feel silenced, as if all of the psychoanalytic gifts he or she can offer have been reduced to empathy. A question or a simple request for clarification can be experienced as a nonempathic response. Some hypervigilant patients scrutinize the therapist for his or her reactions, watching for any indication of inattentiveness or lack of empathy (Gabbard 1998, 2013, 2014), and wait to pounce on a therapist who appears to be losing interest.

The nuances of the countertransference response depend on the particular perspective and subjectivity of the therapist. Some clinicians might feel good about being able to attune and empathize, basking in the countertransference of being a good parent, even imagining themselves as better than the patient's actual mother. Other clinicians may feel manipulated and irritated, drained by their patients and tired of the patients' efforts to get them to say what they want to hear. In other words, the subjectivity of the therapist and the moment in the particular treatment may shape whether the therapist feels like a fount of empathy or a well that is being sucked dry. To make matters more complicated, the same therapist, with the same patient, can feel both ways in the same session.

IDEALIZATION AND MUTUAL ADMIRATION

Some patients regard the therapist as godlike—omnipotent, omniscient, and benevolent. This idealizing transference, as Kohut described it, can be flattering, but it can also lead to a sense of discomfort on the part of the therapist. If the therapist becomes unsettled by the idealization, it can lead him or her to dismantle the idealization prematurely, when in fact some idealization can be helpful in the therapeutic alliance, particularly at the beginning of treatment (Kohut 1971). As therapists, we may have a wish to be idealized, loved, and needed (Finnell 1985), and these patterns may feed our own narcissism and validate our professional skills.

With all admiring patients, and particularly with the high-functioning narcissist, the therapist can find himself or herself engaging in a mutual admiration session with the patient. If the patient is sufficiently entertaining and engaging, the therapist may be "conned" into abdicating a therapeutic relationship and simply enjoying "the show." Although it may be necessary—at least to some extent—for the therapist to join in a modicum of mutual admiration that can build the alliance and foster self-esteem, there are times when fostering the admiration can become problematic. In some cases, a *folie à deux* of sorts may be forged in which the therapist colludes with the patient against looking at real problems in the patient's outside life: although the adoration of the therapist flourishes, the rest of the patient's life deteriorates.

IDENTIFICATION WITH VULNERABILITY

Although there is danger in mutual admiration, there is also a genuine connection that therapists can feel with their narcissistic patients. Despite the data from Tanzilli et al. (2017) and Betan et al. (2005) discussed in the section "Common Patterns of Transference-Counterference With Narcissistic Patients," which showed the most common countertransferences to be predominantly negative, clinicians also can feel a sense of connection and even enthusiasm in working with patients on their issues of self-esteem vulnerability. This positive reaction to narcissistic patients is an underappreciated dimension of work with these individuals that is quite familiar to experienced clinicians. In the example with Mr. E in Chapter 4, "Beginning the Treatment," the therapist felt eager to engage with the patient in an exploration of his feelings that he was facing obscurity and that he had not been able to find his bliss. At times, we clinicians find ourselves impressed at how clearly someone can express his or her wish to be seen in a way that resonates with our own wish to be seen and known. When we hear a patient talk poignantly about the wish to be known or loved, the desire can be compelling and can draw us in. We are more similar to our patients than different. We connect with these patients around the fundamental struggles of being human. Some therapists may come alive with the prospect of helping patients who bring to the therapy their strivings for self-esteem. By contrast, patients who present in a more grandiose, bragging manner likely create less enthusiasm in the therapist's countertransference and more hostility and dread. Many countertransference reports convey a feeling of being "used up" by the patient. When therapist and patient genuinely connect, the therapist may feel useful rather than used up.

ENVY AND COMPETITIVENESS

Klein's (1975) seminal contributions to our understanding of envy have been regarded by Kernberg (1970) as fundamental in patients with narcissistic traits. Envy, competition, and aggression can be felt by both members of the clinical dyad. The therapist may evoke envy in the patient, and similarly, the patient may evoke envy in the therapist, particularly if the patient is highly successful or extraordinarily erudite or clever. With narcissistic patients, Caligor et al. (2015) have described a zero-sum game—in other words, from the perspective of the narcissist, only one person can have status and acclaim, while the other one is automatically relegated to a devalued and demeaned position. To the narcissistic patient, there is a constant comparison going on in the therapy: "I am superior; she is inferior" or vice versa. Hence, the envy may be passed back and forth between patient and therapist. The patient may oscillate between seeing himself as better than the therapist and alternatively seething with envy while imagining that he pales in comparison with the therapist. Similarly, the therapist may find herself enjoying being envied and admired, only to be drawn into envying the patient. Therapists have their own vulnerabilities, and they can be activated when they feel envy of their patient's success, attractiveness, wealth, and so on.

Some narcissistic patients who appear to be highly competitive with their therapist may be flourishing a sense of bravado to cover significant insecurities. Alternatively, they may find it intolerable that the therapist knows more than they do. Narcissists may truly suffer in such situations because in their minds there can be only one "winner" who can have knowledge, success, or power. The therapist must remain attuned to these dynamics and face the likelihood of some form of power struggle with the patient.

CONTEMPT AND DEVALUATION

Therapists often feel deskilled, condescended to, devalued, criticized, and even intimidated by narcissistic patients. In response to being treated with contempt, therapists may have feelings of anger, resentment, and contempt of their own. As Betan et al. (2005) noted in their detailed survey of therapists, the most common countertransference responses to narcissistic patients are likely to be feelings of contempt accompanied by anger and dread. Moreover, therapists may feel defeated in their attempts to be helpful, and the contemptuous patient may rob the therapist of all gratification (Gabbard 2000). Moreover, constantly being berated and demeaned may gradually erode the therapist's sense of confidence in his or her work.

One woman condescendingly asked her therapist, "Isn't there anything in all of those books on your wall that might possibly be of any use to you as you try to help me? Can't you think of even one thing that you learned in all those years of medical school and residency that might make a difference, even a tiny one?" In another case, after listening to his therapist's interpretation, the patient said, "What? That's all you've got? Everything you just said is something I have already told you! I gave it to you! You can't even think of anything original?"

To be sure, all clinicians can succumb to doubt in the face of such contempt. They may wonder if they are truly helping the patient or if the patient is justified in his or her disgust. Clinicians who are at the beginning of their careers may be particularly primed to feel insecure in such moments because their subjective experience of developing a clinical style, expertise, and confidence may be more vulnerable than that of a more experienced clinician. In addition, dynamics of gender, age, race, socioeconomic status, and power may play out in these moments because actions and feelings accompanying contempt carry weight in cultural contexts. For example, a young female therapist may feel differently when being condescended to by a middle-aged man than would a male clinician of similar age to the patient. In addition, certain narcissistic patients will specifically link their contempt to matters of race, ethnicity, or gender, trying to identify the points of maximum vulnerability and provoke an unprofessional response in the therapist (which they can later use against him or her).

OMNIPOTENT CONTROL

As noted in Chapter 3 in our discussion of modes of relatedness, attempting to control what someone else feels, says, or does is a pervasive tactic of narcissistic patients. In their view, this omnipotent control gives them the upper hand in the therapeutic encounter and defends against any surprise or humiliation. Some patients come in with a long list on a notepad or a smartphone and stick to it at all costs, despite any attempt on the part of the therapist to shift the conversation to another topic. The hypervigilant patient may exert control over the therapist by keeping his or her eyes glued to the therapist and scrutinizing every shift in weight, clearing of the throat, raising of an eyebrow, or concealed yawn in an effort to ferret out any subtle signs of potential boredom, disagreement, disapproval, faulty attunement, or negative judgment. As noted previously, some patients can tolerate only empathy and will try to "sniff out" all other forms of reaction and shame the therapist for not responding in the "proper way" (Gabbard 2013).

Symington (1990) has noted that in some patients, projective identification itself is an attempt to control the therapist's freedom of thought. Hence, the patient's omnipotent control can make it difficult for the therapist to think clearly or even to think at all. The therapist may feel like an excluded outsider who is allowed only a narrow range of thoughts and words. As a result of feeling disconnected and remote, the therapist may engage in a competition-fueled challenge in which he reasserts his voice into the therapeutic dialogue. In so doing, the therapist may miss an opportunity to reflect on the countertransference as a way of understanding the patient's fear of what the therapist may say. When therapists feel controlled in this manner, they can begin to empathize with the deep-seated terror in narcissistic patients about the potential for others to hurt them. They are convinced that if they cannot control every move, every word, and every thought of those who matter to them, they will be abandoned or rejected.

As a result of feeling treated like a "function," the therapist may develop a feeling of loneliness in the room. The lack of interpersonal mutuality and exchange can leave the therapist feeling isolated. Another possibility is that the therapist can become fed up with the patient's demands and reply with an obstinate refusal to meet any of the patient's requests. In so doing, the therapist misses the opportunity for necessary affirmation and gratification of some of the patient's needs and wishes.

Although we have suggested some common transference-countertransference constellations found in narcissistic patients, we must close by acknowledging that there are a host of other paradigms that grow out of the meetings of two minds in the crucible of the consulting room. A cornerstone of intersubjective thought is that the interaction of two separate subjectivities will inevitably create unexpected experiences in addition to the familiar interactions that have haunted the patient (and the therapist) throughout life.

REFERENCES

Benjamin J: Beyond Doer and Done to: Recognition Theory, Intersubjectivity, and the Third. New York, Routledge, 2018

Betan E, Heim AK, Zittel Conklin C, et al: Countertransference phenomena and personality pathology in clinical practice: an empirical investigation. Am J Psychiatry 162(5):890–898, 2005 15863790

Brenner D: The Mind in Conflict. New York, International Universities Press, 1982

Caligor E, Levy KN, Yeomans FE: Narcissistic personality disorder: diagnostic and clinical challenges. Am J Psychiatry 172(5):415–422, 2015 25930131

Carpy DV: Tolerating the countertransference: a mutative process. Int J Psychoanal 70(Pt 2):287–294, 1989 2753609

Cooper AM: The narcissistic-masochistic character. Psychiatr Ann 39(10):904–912, 2009

Dombek K: The Selfishness of Others: An Essay on the Fear of Narcissism. New York, Farrar, Straus, and Giroux, 2016

Fairbairn WRD: Endopsychic structure considered in terms of object-relationships (1944), in Psychoanalytic Studies of the Personality. London, Routledge and Kegan Paul, 1952, pp 82–132

Finnell JS: Narcissistic problems in analysts. Int J Psychoanal 66(4):433–445, 1985

Freud S: The future prospects for psycho-analytic therapy (1910), in The Standard Edition of the Complete Works of Sigmund Freud, Vol 11. Translated and edited by Strachey J. London, Hogarth, 1957, pp 139–151

Freud S: On narcissism: an introduction (1914), in The Standard Edition of the Complete Works of Sigmund Freud, Vol 14. Translated and edited by Strachey J. London, Hogarth, 1963, pp 67–102

Gabbard GO: Two subtypes of narcissistic personality disorder. Bull Menninger Clin 53(6):527–532, 1989 2819295

Gabbard GO: Transference and countertransference in the treatment of narcissistic patients, in Disorders of Narcissism: Diagnostic, Clinical and Empirical Implications. Edited by Ronningstam EF. Washington, DC, American Psychiatric Press, 1998, pp. 125–146

Gabbard GO: On gratitude and gratification. J Am Psychoanal Assoc 48(3):697–716, 2000 11059393

Gabbard GO: Countertransference issues in the treatment of pathological narcissism, in Understanding and Treating Pathological Narcissism. Edited by Ogrodniczuk JS. Washington DC, American Psychological Association, 2013, pp 207–217

Gabbard GO: Psychodynamic Psychiatry in Clinical Practice, 5th Edition. Arlington, VA, American Psychiatric Publishing, 2014

Gabbard GO, Crisp-Han H: The many faces of narcissism. World Psychiatry 15(2):115–116, 2016 27265694

Gabbard GO, Ogden TH: On becoming a psychoanalyst. Int J Psychoanal 90(2):311–327, 2009 19382962

Heimann P: On counter-transference. Int J Psychoanal 31:81–84, 1950

Kernberg OF: Factors in the psychoanalytic treatment of narcissistic personalities. J Am Psychoanal Assoc 18(1):51–85, 1970 5451020

Kernberg OF: Further contributions to the treatment of narcissistic personalities. Int J Psychoanal 55(2):215–247, 1974 4448592

Kernberg OF: Borderline Conditions and Pathological Narcissism. New York, Jason Aronson, 1975

Kernberg OF: An overview of the treatment of severe narcissistic pathology. Int J Psychoanal 95(5):865–888, 2014 24902768

Klein M: Notes on some schizoid mechanisms (1946), in Envy and Gratitude and Other Works, 1946–1963. New York, Free Press, 1975, pp 1–24

Kohut H: The Analysis of the Self: A Systematic Approach to the Psychoanalytic Treatment of Narcissistic Personality Disorders. New York, International Universities Press, 1971

Kohut H: The Restoration of the Self. New York, International Universities Press, 1977

Kohut H: How Does Analysis Cure? Edited by Goldberg A. Chicago, IL, University of Chicago Press, 1984

Liberman DM: Kohut's self psychology approach to treating pathological narcissism, in Understanding and Treating Pathological Narcissism. Edited by Ogrodniczuk JS. Washington, DC, American Psychological Association, 2013, pp 253–268

Masterson J: The Narcissistic and Borderline Conditions. New York, Brunnere/Mazel, 1981

Ogden TH: On projective identification. Int J Psychoanal 60(Pt 3):357–373, 1979 533737

Ogden TH: Projective Identification and Psychotherapeutic Technique. New York, Jason Aronson, 1982

Ogden TH: Why read Fairbairn? Int J Psychoanal 91(1):101–118, 2010 20433477

Ringstrom P: Cultivating the improvisational in psychoanalytic treatment. Psychoanal Dialogues 11(5):727–754, 2001

Rosen IC: The wish to be hated: Richard III's villainy in pursuit of the bad-enough object. J Am Psychoanal Assoc 61(6):1175–1195, 2013 24304519

Russ E, Shedler J, Bradley R, et al: Refining the construct of narcissistic personality disorder: diagnostic criteria and subtypes. Am J Psychiatry 165(11):1473–1481, 2008 18708489

Steiner J: Seeing and being seen: narcissistic pride and narcissistic humiliation. Int J Psychoanal 87(Pt 4):939–951, 2006 16877245

Symington N: The possibility of human freedom and its transmission (with particular reference to the thought of Bion). Int J Psychoanal 71(Pt 1):95–106, 1990 2332301

Tanzilli A, Muzi L, Ronningstam E, et al: Countertransference when working with narcissistic personality disorder: An empirical investigation. Psychotherapy (Chic) 54(2):184–194, 2017 28581327

Winnicott DW: Hate in the countertransference. Int J Psychoanal 30:69–74, 1949

Winnicott DW: Ego distortion in terms of true and false self (1960), in The Maturational Processes and the Facilitating Environment. New York, International Universities Press, 1965, pp 140–152

6

Tailoring the Treatment to the Patient

Any discussion involving the treatment of narcissistic personality disorder (NPD) must acknowledge the fact that we have no randomized controlled studies to guide us. Neither do we have naturalistic treatment studies that follow the course of patients over time. Ogrodniczuk (2013) notes that "the limited research regarding the treatment of pathological narcissism is a significant concern, and is perhaps surprising given the amount of attention paid to narcissism in clinical literature" (p. 6). This absence of systematic treatment research is striking in light of the fact that surveys have shown that as many as 25% of outpatients in psychotherapy have the diagnosis of NPD (Doidge et al. 2002). Moreover, clinicians clamored for the inclusion of NPD in DSM-5 (American Psychiatric Association 2013) when it appeared that it might disappear from the official diagnostic nomenclature.

In the absence of data from randomized controlled trials, treatment for NPD has been driven by psychoanalytic theory for several decades. The major controversy has been the clash between the writings of Kohut (1971, 1977) and Kernberg (1975, 1984), as described in previous chapters. Despite their differences, Kohut and Kernberg both approached the narcissistic patient as someone who requires analysis or high-frequency psychoanalytic psychotherapy.

Empathy was the cornerstone of technique for Kohut, who argued that therapists need to empathize with the patient's attempts to activate a failed parental relationship. He saw the major action in the treatment as an attempt by the patient to coerce the therapist into meeting the patient's need for affirmation (mirror transference), for idealization (idealizing transference), or for being like the therapist (twinship transference). He felt that the emergence of these three selfobject transferences should not be prematurely interpreted. He stressed that empathizing with the patient as a victim of the empathic failures of others does not imply a predominantly supportive technique. Rather, Kohut stressed that the analyst or therapist should *interpret*—rather than gratify—the patient's yearning to be soothed.

By contrast, Kernberg stressed that the therapist must focus on envy and how it prevents the patient from receiving or acknowledging help. He also emphasized confronting the aggression and competitiveness in the patient. He felt it was necessary for the analyst or therapist to systematically examine both positive and negative transference developments. In addition, he made it clear that although psychoanalysis is generally the treatment of choice for NPD, overtly borderline functioning in narcissistic patients is a contraindication for psychoanalysis. In such cases, he recommended expressive psychotherapy (Kernberg 2010).

Kernberg's approach to treating borderline personality disorder (BPD) has evolved into a systematic twice-weekly psychodynamic psychotherapy commonly referred to as *transference-focused psychotherapy* (TFP; Caligor et al. 2007; Clarkin et al. 2006). Following Kernberg's theoretical framework, the ultimate goal is to promote integration of the unintegrated representations of self and others and assist the patient in tolerating negative effects such as aggression, envy, and anxiety. In addition, the treatment focuses on interpersonal relationships and work functioning such that both are improved as part of the patient's overall functioning. There are now two well-controlled randomized clinical trials that demonstrate the effectiveness of TFP with BPD (Clarkin et al. 2007; Doering et al. 2010).

The adaptation of TFP to narcissistic patients is based on Kernberg's view that NPD is characterized by an underlying borderline personality organization similar to that of the patient with BPD. The treatment process in TFP with narcissistic patients is similar to the manner in which it is conducted with borderline patients; that is, the therapist tracks the emergence of the split-off self and object configurations and actively interprets them (Stern et al. 2013). One dyadic configuration that is common in narcissistic patients is a grandiose and independent self in relation to a devalued and dependent other. These respective roles can, of course, be projected onto the therapist and then re-introjected by the patient in a moment-to-moment ongoing process.

Transference interpretation is central to TFP. It begins with a request for clarification regarding the patient's objective experience, followed by a confrontation of an apparent contradiction in the patient's communication, and finally an interpretation that links what is going on in the transference to unconscious determinants within the patient. Clinical experience teaches us that although some narcissistic patients respond favorably to transference interpretation, others do not. In the absence of systematic controlled studies, one must exercise caution about the use of transference interpretation in patients with narcissistic organizations. In this context it is useful to review what we know from research regarding the use of transference interpretation in general.

THE ROLE OF TRANSFERENCE INTERPRETATION

Although transference interpretation has long been valorized as the ultimate intervention in psychoanalytically oriented treatments, the recent discourse among psychoanalysts and psychotherapy researchers has raised questions about that emphasis. Studies of the long-term effects of transference work have actually shown mixed results. In a review of the subject, Høglend and Gabbard (2012) noted that some research found no correlations or weak correlations between transference interpretation and outcomes, whereas some others found negative associations, and still others found positive associations. In one study reviewed, a subsample of patients with high levels of object relations scores found negative correlations between the number of transference interpretations and outcomes (Piper et al. 1999). Connolly et al. (1999) found that patients with poor interpersonal functioning improved less with even as little as two or fewer transference interpretations per session. Ogrodniczuk et al. (1999) found that in patients with low quality of object relations, there were negative correlations between moderate frequency of transference interpretations (two to four per session) and both outcome and alliance.

A particularly influential study on transference interpretation in once-weekly psychotherapy was conducted by Høglend et al. (2006). In this investigation, a randomized controlled trial of 12 months of dynamic psychotherapy, 100 outpatients were randomly assigned either to a group using transference interpretation or to a group that did not use transference interpretation. The group receiving transference interpretations had moderate levels of one to three per session. Patients with impaired object relations benefited more from therapies using transference interpretation than those without transference interpretation. The investigators found that this effect was sustained at a 3-year follow-up.

In a subsequent report, Høglend et al. (2011) examined the effects of transference work in the context of therapeutic alliance and quality of object relations in more detail. They found that in patients with a strong alliance and higher levels of object relations, the specific effect of transference work tended to be smaller and only marginally significant. Transference work had a stronger specific effect for patients with low quality of object relations scale scores within the context of a weak alliance.

One implication of this finding is that transference work may be particularly important with those patients who have difficulties establishing stable and fulfilling relationships. Patients with high levels of object relations may not require a good deal of transference interpretation. On the other hand, those with difficulties in relationships may benefit from a careful interpretation and understanding of the anxieties in the here-and-now relationship with the therapist.

Although NPD was not the primary focus of Høglend's research, one can infer from this research that some narcissistically disturbed patients may benefit from examination of the transference in detail. On the other hand, clinicians know that some narcissistic patients feel that interpretation of the transference is jarring. They may feel that they are being blamed for their difficulties or criticized by the therapist (a manifestation of their hypersensitivity). Narcissistic patients often feel that they are sharing legitimate responses to real behaviors or attitudes of the therapist and can feel hurt and angry about being "pathologized."

> Mr. M is a 46-year-old executive in a moderately successful company who came to treatment because he felt his skills and expertise were not sufficiently noted in the workplace. He felt irritable, somewhat depressed, and at odds with his wife, who he felt was insufficiently sym-

pathetic to his plight at the office. He told his therapist that this lack of appreciation for the way he got treated went all the way back to his parents. He bitterly recounted how when he was bullied at school, he would come home and tell his dad about it. His dad's only response was to taunt him by saying, "Complain, complain, complain." He told the therapist in great detail about instances at work where he had been ridiculed, ignored, belittled, and overlooked while people of lesser talents and intelligence were promoted. In his first three sessions with his therapist, he cataloged numerous incidents that featured situations in which others misunderstood him, and the therapist listened sympathetically.

In the fourth session, the therapist raised a question with Mr. M: "Is there anything that you might be doing to contribute to the situation?" Mr. M seemed hurt and was silent for a moment. Then he said, "I am trying to explain to you something important about the dog-eat-dog world I live in, but I feel like you are not really hearing me and are trying to make it all my fault." After a pause he said, "I don't feel like saying anything now." The therapist wondered out loud, "I guess I'm probably sounding like your dad right now." Mr. M became indignant at this point and said, "No, that's not true. You really aren't hearing me because you are blaming me instead of the outrageous people I work with." The therapist responded by saying, "Then tell me more about these people so I'll gain a better understanding of them." He made a choice to not continue pushing his point in the fourth session when Mr. M clearly was indicating that the transference interpretation was not welcome. Moreover, he felt that he needed to establish a more solid therapeutic alliance before another foray into transference work.

Although we do not have systematic data about the specific responses of patients with NPD to transference interpretation, a process study of BPD (Gabbard et al. 1994) provides some data that may be relevant to the issues under consideration. In this investigation, three patients diagnosed with BPD were in long-term dynamic therapy with experienced psychoanalytic therapists. Using tape recordings of sessions, the researchers examined upward and downward shifts in the collaboration between patient and therapist (as an indicator of the therapeutic alliance) following transference interpretations. They found that the three patients responded quite differently to transference interventions. In one patient, only 29% of all upward shifts in collaboration were linked to transference work. In the second patient, 63% of upward shifts were linked to transference work, and in the third, 81% of the upward shift followed transference comments. The researchers concluded that transference interpretations were found to have a greater impact, *both* positive and negative, on the therapeutic alliance, which suggested that transference interpretation is a high-risk, high-gain enterprise.

Clinical work with narcissistic patients has not been studied as vigorously, but it is certainly true that transference interpretation may have both highly positive and highly negative effects with this population. In fact, although Kohut insisted that his technical approach did not depart radically from classical psychoanalytic technique and was focused on interpreting the transference, his suggestions to supervisees appear to reflect departures from classical transference interpretation (Miller 1985). Kohut advised some analysts he was supervising to take the analytic material in a "straight manner" just as the patient experienced it rather than looking at what was underneath the manifest content. In so doing, he suggested, one did not repeat the empathic failures of the parents, which often involved an attempt to convince a child that his or her actual feelings are *different* from those the child describes.

Further study of the audiotaped recordings in the Gabbard et al. (1994) study revealed that high-gain transference interpretations were generally preceded by a series of interventions that were closer to the supportive end of the expressive-supportive continuum, including empathic validation, clarification, advice and praise, and encouragement to elaborate. Paving the way for transference interpretation with borderline patients appears to create a sense of a holding environment where the patient can hear the interpretation in a more receptive space. The same preparatory phase may be necessary when dealing with narcissistic patients. Indeed, TFP has structured the interpretive approach to NPD patients so that a series of interventions is provided in which the interventions build on one another before the therapist offers an interpretation proper (Stern et al. 2013).

One way to understand that both Kernberg and Kohut reported success in their respective treatments is to note that Kohut's sample may have been different from Kernberg's. It is possible that Kohut treated a greater number of vulnerable, hypervigilant narcissists compared with Kernberg's cohort. Moreover, the two clinicians may have had different views of what constitutes a positive outcome.

Another key point in discerning the optimal technique with narcissistic patients is that the specific characteristics of the individual must be taken into account. A generic diagnostic category such as NPD falls short of stipulating how therapists should adjust their approach to the idiosyncrasies of the patient. With oblivious patients who hold forth in the session in a manner that makes the therapist feel marginalized, the impact of transference interpretation may be almost imperceptible. The patient may experience the clinician's comment as an annoying interruption or a distraction and go right on as if nothing had been said. In such situations, a transference interpretation may be a no risk, no gain intervention.

On the other hand, a hypervigilant patient may have a devastating response to a comment that seems extraordinarily benign to the therapist:

> Ms. N is an attorney who was seeing Dr. O in twice-weekly psychotherapy that focused heavily on her experiences of being slighted by the paralegals (all females) with whom she worked. She felt she was not respected and was repeatedly challenged by them in her daily work. When discussing the paralegals, she frequently said, "Where did they get their law degree?" She spent many sessions chronicling her list of grievances, and as she spoke, she would study the face of Dr. O to discern his reaction to what she was saying. At one point, Dr. O attempted to make an empathic comment by saying, "I can appreciate how you must feel." Ms. N reacted with scorn and disbelief: "No, I don't believe you can. Number 1, you're a man. Number 2, you weren't there! You can't possibly know what it is like."

One would have to conclude that the role of transference interpretation in a particular treatment is an ongoing project. Trial and error will gradually shed some light on its usefulness. Friedman (2002) has cautioned that interpretive work within the transference carries with it the potential to shock or annoy the patient because it is experienced as an implicit assault on the entrenched beliefs of the patient. The timing of such interventions is highly relevant, and the idiosyncratic features of the patient are of great importance. Creating a holding environment that builds a therapeutic alliance with the patient may be essential. Finally, one is wise to postpone transference interpretation until the accumulated evidence for one's formulation is substantial.

TAILORING THE THERAPY TO THE PATIENT

In light of the limited research on the role of transference interpretation, one needs to move slowly during the assessment phase with a new patient to determine the optimal approach. One can offer a trial interpretation involving transference issues and note how the patient responds. This strategy was illustrated in the case of Mr. M earlier. The therapist made a foray into transference work and then backed off when he realized that Mr. M was narcissistically wounded by his comment.

In determining whether or not the patient can use an analytic or highly expressive psychotherapy, the therapist must consider other variables in addition to response to transference interventions. Although there has been a tradition of identifying psychoanalysis as the treatment of choice for patients with NPD, there is now a broad consensus that this view is overstated. Some patients do better with an expressive psychotherapy in which they are sitting up. Ronningstam (2014) noted that although the use of the couch in formal psychoanalysis may improve awareness of the self, it also

> protects the patients and prevents them from accessing and addressing certain areas of pathological narcissistic patterns. In other words, deeper aspects of a patient's self-sustaining regulation may be "contained" or "out of reach" in the absence of face-to-face interaction, leading to partial or pseudo progress or stalemates with lack of deeper characterological changes. (p. 1,082)

Ronningstam noted that TFP is useful for those patients who need face-to-face work with full eye contact to counterbalance detachment and emotional disengagement. In addition, some patients who are being seen in three- or four-times-weekly psychoanalysis might actually do better sitting up.

Whether one is considering psychoanalysis or psychoanalytic psychotherapy, the capacity for self-reflectiveness and psychological mindedness is extraordinarily important for expressive work. One measure of this capacity is the ability to draw analogies between what happens in one relationship and what happens in another. Some degree of honesty and integrity, as opposed to corruption and deceptiveness, also is necessary for a highly expressive treatment. Strong motivation to understand oneself is another indication. Finally, a capacity for affect tolerance bodes well for psychoanalysis proper or a highly psychoanalytic therapy. Among narcissistic patients, there is considerable variability in their capacity to use transference work. Some seem to work better with an extratransference focus. Similarly, some will respond more favorably to an approach that deemphasizes interpretation.

Therapists should keep in mind the time-honored notion of an expressive-supportive continuum when they are attempting to tailor the therapy to the patient (See Figure 6–1).

Most therapies involve moving back and forth across this continuum, using interventions that involve confrontation and interpretation when possible and offering empathic validation and advice when necessary. The therapist has to be attuned to the patient's frame of mind. Timing is everything. This basic premise is especially true with narcissistic patients because their sense of well-being is highly influenced by the context in which they find themselves. As noted in Chapter 1, "Narcissism and Its Discontents," an apparently self-confident grandiose narcissist can fall apart and be desperately helpless when receiving a critical comment or a slight from a valued person in his or her life. In this way the patient "supervises" the therapist.

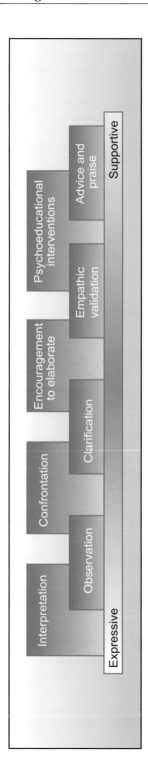

Figure 6–1. An expressive-supportive continuum of interventions.

Source. Reprinted from Gabbard GO: *Long-Term Psychodynamic Psychotherapy: A Basic Text*, 3rd Edition (Core Competencies in Psychotherapy). Arlington, VA, American Psychiatric Association Publishing, 2017. Copyright © American Psychiatric Association Publishing. Used with permission.

In his Italian seminars, Wilford Bion (2005) emphasized that theory must never be privileged over direct clinical observation. Patients, after all, do not come to analysis because they suffer from a provocative theory:

> We could say that there is one collaborator we have in analysis on whom we can rely because he behaves as if he really had a mind and because he thought that somebody not himself could help. In short, the most important assistance that a psychoanalyst is likely to get is not from his analyst, or supervisor or teacher, or the books that he can read, but from his patient. The patient—and only the patient—knows what it feels like to be him or her. (Bion 2005, p. 3)

TREATMENT PLANNING

Much of the writing on narcissistic patients is geared to the most intensive form of treatment, usually psychoanalysis or psychoanalytic psychotherapy that takes place multiple times per week. However, in an era when fees have gone up and insurance support has gone down, many narcissistic patients find it difficult to afford the treatment that might provide the most optimal outcome. Hence, treatments of a frequency of two to four times per week are often beyond the grasp of the patient who is seeking help.

Another limitation on frequency is lack of motivation to come more than once per week. As noted in Chapter 4, "Beginning the Treatment," many narcissistic patients present themselves as busy professionals who can barely find an hour in their schedule each week to come for treatment. Although this presentation can be dealt with over time as anxiety about becoming dependent on a therapist or fear of being exposed to shame and humiliation, some patients may hold to this position tenaciously. Therapists may need to accommodate to the once-weekly request for an extended period of time to build a therapeutic alliance with the patient and ultimately soften the patient's resistance so he or she is willing to come more frequently.

Regardless of the reason for settling on once-weekly therapy, therapists can be encouraged by the previously mentioned randomized controlled trial by Høglend and colleagues (Høglend and Gabbard 2012; Høglend et al. 2006). As noted in the section "The Role of Transference Interpretations," patients with more disturbed object relations showed benefit from transference interpretations. It is useful in this context to clarify that the investigators used a broader set of techniques under the heading of transference than the strict psychoanalytic version of transference *interpretation*. The following specific techniques were prescribed for the group with transference focus:

(1) the therapist was to address transactions in the patient-therapist relationship; (2) the therapist was to encourage exploration of thoughts and feelings about the therapy and therapist; (3) the therapist was to include himself explicitly in interpretative linking of dynamic elements (conflicts), direct manifestations of transference, allusions to the transference, and repercussions on the transference by high-therapist activity; (4) the therapist was to encourage the patient to discuss how he or she believed the therapist might feel or think about him or her; (5) the therapist was to interpret repetitive interpersonal patterns (including genetic interpretations) and link these patterns to transactions between the patient and the therapist. (Høglend et al. 2006, p. 1,741)

When all five of these techniques are considered, one might think of the approach as transference work that includes transference exploration as well as interpretation proper. In other words, some of the elements involve preparatory work for interpretation that focuses to some extent on the relationship between patient and therapist, as described earlier in the section "The Role of Transference Interpretation." Hence, an approach to a once-weekly patient that includes this broader version of transference work may be helpful in improving the object relations of the patient while preparing him or her for more intensive treatment. Even those who continue at a frequency of once weekly may well benefit.

A therapy that focuses on mentalization may also be useful for patients with NPD. As noted in Chapter 3, "Modes of Relatedness," narcissistic patients may have a good deal of difficulty discerning what is going on inside another person's mind. Bateman and Fonagy (2012) noted that NPD patients may have a fairly well-developed self-focus but an extremely limited grasp of what others are feeling. Mentalization-based therapy (MBT) is well developed for BPD and was shown to be superior to structured clinical management in a randomized controlled trial (Bateman and Fonagy 2009). Substantial improvements were noted on interpersonal measures, social adjustment, mood, and need for hospitalization.

MBT lies somewhere between TFP and supportive therapy. The aims of MBT are more modest than those of TFP. It does not attempt to achieve structural personality change. Rather, it is designed to promote a mentalizing attitude to problems and relationships and to help the patient become more curious about his or her own mental states and those of others (Bateman and Fonagy 2012). Although MBT does not emphasize transference interpretation, it encourages therapists to mentalize the transference as part of the therapy. It should be noted in this regard that with BPD patients, TFP also appears to improve reflective function and thus enhance the mentalizing capacity of patients (Levy et al. 2006).

Certain patients who are narcissistically organized can tolerate only empathic comments that demonstrate the therapist's understanding and validation of how they feel. Even a gentle clarification or confrontation can sometimes cause a fragmented or angry reaction in the patient. Nevertheless, the therapist may become a key source of comfort, empathy, and acceptance. In our experience, some patients do well over time as long as they continue to have this availability of a humane therapist who listens carefully to them and takes seriously what they say. Because of this support, some narcissistic patients are able to maintain a stable equilibrium so they can function in their societal role.

A subgroup of narcissistic patients cannot tolerate coming to therapy weekly because the intensity of the relationship creates too much anxiety. They may opt for an appointment every 2 or 3 weeks. Some may "officially" be in weekly therapy but regularly miss or "forget" sessions such that they are seen only once or twice a month. There are others who wish to come anywhere from once a month to once every 3 or 4 months. In such cases, the therapist is faced with "managing" the patient as best as possible with the limitations imposed by the patient. Some patients need to gradually build up to a weekly or twice-weekly therapy because they do not feel it is "safe" to come more often. Their anxiety about closeness outside the therapy is transferred to the relationship within the therapy.

There is an unfortunate and long-standing tradition of denigrating supportive psychotherapy in our field. A common error made by both beginning and experienced psychodynamic therapists is to overestimate the capacity of the patient to use insight brought about by interpretation. In the Menninger Foundation Psychotherapy Research Project, Wallerstein (1986) followed 42 patients over a period of 30 years. Many of these patients benefited because the psychotherapists shifted gears in the course of the therapy. The therapists had typically begun with the expectation of an interpretive or expressive reproach only to find that the patient had greater deficits in ego capacity than previously recognized. When therapists shifted to the more supportive end of the continuum, some of these patients had reasonably good outcomes.

We have little research to guide us on the use of supportive psychotherapy with narcissistic patients. However, a randomized controlled trial of long-term therapies for patients with BPD (Clarkin et al. 2007; Levy et al. 2006) provides some data that may be relevant to NPD. The study involved a comparison of TFP, dialectical behavior therapy, and supportive therapy, all of which lasted 1 year. Ninety patients were randomly assigned to one of the three groups. All three groups showed similar levels of improvement, but the TFP patients showed greater increases in mentalization as measured by reflective functioning and movement in the direction of more secure attachment. A major finding regarding supportive psychotherapy, however, was that it appeared to improve depression, anxiety, global functioning, social adjustment, impulsivity, and anger.

Carsky (2013) defined the essence of this modality as involving the provision of validation, emotional support, praise, and problem solving to maintain a therapeutic relationship characterized by a preponderance of positive over negative transference. The therapist specifically focuses on creating an atmosphere free of narcissistic injury. Hence, although no systematic research exists on supportive therapy of narcissistic patients, clinicians find that there is a large subgroup of such patients who cannot tolerate a more expressive approach to the transference. Carsky clarified that the therapist should avoid explicit interpretation of transference fantasy while at the same time using awareness of transference as a way of monitoring the patient's self-esteem. Other elements of supportive therapy include the growth of identity through modeling by the therapist, increasing the awareness and tolerance of affect, and monitoring the frame (Carsky 2013).

Kernberg (1975) reviewed the results of the Psychotherapy Research Project of the Menninger Foundation and noted that supportive therapy was useful with a subgroup of patients in the study. He concluded that patients with severe narcissistic character structure combined with overt borderline functioning could be treated successfully with a purely supportive approach. In Chapter 7, "Specific Treatment Strategies," we describe a supportive strategy for those narcissistic patients who do not seem able to use psychotherapy to make significant changes.

GROUP PSYCHOTHERAPY

Psychodynamic group psychotherapy is another useful modality for many narcissistic patients. It is probably most effective when used in conjunction with individual psychotherapy so that the patient's reaction to events in the group therapy can be processed within the context of a one-to-one therapeutic relationship (Ronningstam 2014). However, group therapy may be a double-edged sword for patients with NPD. On the one hand, they may enjoy the idea of having an audience. On the other hand, they may resent the fact that other people take some of the therapist's attention and time away from them. It is not uncommon for narcissistic patients to walk out of a group after they have finished what they wanted to say, unconcerned about what others may need to share. With hypervigilant narcissists, the referral itself may be experienced as a rejection by the therapist, whom they view as not interested in them. Ogrodniczuk et al. (2014) observed that the narcissist's hunger for admiration, lack of empathy, and sense of entitlement may alienate other members of the group. Some narcissists will view group psychotherapy as a place where their specialness and uniqueness will not be recognized. They may function as "the doctor's assistant," remarking on the pathology of the other people of the group while denying their own (Wong 1979).

The other edge of the double-edged sword is that the situation is ideally suited for narcissistic patients to confront the unavoidable fact that others have needs and that they themselves cannot always be the center of attention. Moreover, group therapy may be the only setting where other people will speak directly to how the patient's character traits affect them. Group psychotherapy may also serve to dilute intense negative transferences. Other patients may be able to confront a narcissistic patient who devalues the therapist or, on the other hand, idealizes the therapist. Most experts suggest that it is preferable to have only one narcissistic patient at a time in a heterogeneous group or the patient's demandingness may overwhelm the other members and cause them to leave. One advantage, of course, is that the group therapy fee may be much lower and affordable for patients who are not able to pay the full fee of individual treatment.

MBT integrates individual and group therapy (Bateman and Fonagy 2012). Hence, formal studies of MBT have measured both treatments as part of a conjoint therapy. In some cases, the same therapist conducts both the individual therapy and the group therapy, whereas in others, two different therapists are used. Although data on NPD patients in this kind of conjoint therapy are lacking, some clinicians report that the group modality can enhance the mentalizing process, both for inpatients and for outpatients.

COUPLES AND FAMILY THERAPY

Some narcissistic patients who are in psychoanalysis or individual psychotherapy may be consistently attending sessions and may be motivated to learn more about themselves. The relationship with the analyst or therapist may be characterized by a reasonably good therapeutic alliance, but problems with the patient's spouse or partner continue. Particular relational paradigms that are largely based in unconscious internal object relations may surface only with the spouse or partner, whereas others are apparent in the transference to the treater. Couples therapy (conducted by a different therapist) may be valuable in these situations so that the particular impasses that appear in the couple's relationship can emerge fully and be examined in the context of both partners. The modes of relatedness causing the interpersonal problems in the marriage or partnership may have been obscured by the way the patient presented himself or herself in individual treatment.

As noted in Chapter 1, some patients with NPD or narcissistic traits may not appear to be distressed by their difficulties but may cause considerable distress in others. Hence, a common scenario is that a spouse or partner will tell the narcissist that he or she "must get treatment or else." The reluctant patient may then dutifully go to see a therapist to head off a divorce or to placate an angry spouse. On arrival, the patients in this situation may present themselves as having no idea why they are there or what they need to work on. They may instead blame the spouse or partner for being hypersensitive and "the one with the real problem." In some cases, this externalization or projective disavowal can be confronted by the therapist such that the patient becomes more self-reflective. In other situations, the patient is fairly refractory to any suggestion that he or she may be responsible for difficulties in the marriage or relationship. In such situations, couples therapy may be the preferred modality because the person who is distressed is there as a source of information about the designated patient's problems.

Bringing a spouse or partner into the consulting room offers an opportunity to help a nonmentalizing patient begin to appreciate how he or she makes others feel. The therapist can bring out the significant other's frustration and exasperation with not feeling understood or appreciated. With a neutral third party present, the patient must hear about his or her shortcomings from someone who is intimately familiar with the typical ways of relating that have caused the patient to have difficulties. When the narcissistic partner dismisses the observations of the significant other, the therapist can in fact hold the patient's feet to the fire and insist that attention must be paid to these concerns. Over time, the narcissistic patient's difficulty in mentalizing can be addressed by encouraging appreciation of the spouse or partner's experience of living with someone who does not seem to take an interest in how others feel in his or her presence. The couple's therapist can actively encourage the narcissistic patient to inquire about the impact he or she is having on the spouse or partner. The patient must then listen attentively while feedback is provided about that impact and how the other person thinks and feels. This procedure may go a long way toward educating the narcissist about what he or she has been systematically avoiding as part of the narcissistic isolation that has pervaded his or her life.

The introduction of a family member into this discussion touches on another possibility: family therapy in the treatment of narcissistic patients. This modality is probably underutilized for narcissistic patients, and the reasons for that are not entirely clear. In contrast, the approach to BPD often includes a strong family component that incorporates a psychoeducational program for both patient and family (Gunderson and Hoffman 2005). One reason that this component has been incorporated is that there is a large body of research to draw from in the understanding and treatment of BPD. For example, the biological factors at work in BPD are better understood than those related to NPD. In addition, sophisticated research has led to empirically validated psychotherapies that have been shown to improve BPD. Pharmacology research showing how specific medications can relieve both cognitive and affective symptoms of BPD are also part of a typical psychoeducational program.

By contrast, such data are not available for NPD. Moreover, there is a greater stigma attached to the term *narcissistic* than to the term *borderline*. The extensive neurobiological research on BPD also removes it from blaming the patient or the family for bad behavior. The current thinking about BPD is that neurobiological vulnerability interacts with environmental stressors. That kind of biological research is not available for NPD, and it is much easier for families to blame the parents or the patients for the condition. Hence, there has not been a systematic approach to developing family involvement with NPD as there is with BPD.

Nonetheless, family work may be extremely helpful when the patient is a young adult who is a "failure to launch," remaining dependent on the parents rather than achieving such milestones as moving out and acquiring a job. Such individuals manifest some version of an unfulfilled potential. They may have a sense of entitlement to a glamorous job but feel that they should not have to undergo rigorous education or training to prepare themselves for the job market. They may also be an embarrassment to their parents, who have a combination of shame for their parental failures and anger at their child. These young adults often are brought to a mental health professional to be "fixed." In most cases, however, a family process, by itself or in conjunction with individual therapy, may be necessary for change to take place. Often, there is a history of overvaluation of the child associated with expectations that are excessive and daunting for the young adult. Moreover, the parents may have enabled the son or daughter's dependent state by taking over tasks—writing college papers, filling out job applications—that seem to overwhelm the young adult child. Family treatment may get the family "unstuck" and mobilized to develop a plan. A clinician working with the family can focus on the difference between helping in a way that promotes further dependency and helping in a manner that allows the young adult to struggle and develop some form of active mastery over his or her dilemma.

Adult children in this situation may also be deriving unconscious or conscious pleasure from thwarting their parents' vision of who they should be. They may have deeply resented the pressure to achieve and excel as a narcissistic extension of the parents. Another possibility is that they have cognitive problems that have gone undiagnosed or a major psychiatric disorder about which the family is in denial. In other words, they may truly be limited, but the parents are blind to that limitation. Finally, the adult child may simply have a different agenda for his or her life, and the parents may require help to mourn the loss of their vision for their son or daughter. The narcissism may reside in the parents' grandiose expectations rather than in the child. In any case, working with the family system instead of a single individual is often essential in such cases.

INPATIENT AND INTENSIVE OUTPATIENT TREATMENT

Although most of the literature on the treatment of narcissistic patients focuses on outpatient therapy or analysis, more structured inpatient or intensive outpatient treatment may be necessary. For instance, suicidal patients may require round-the-clock observation because of their risk for impulsive or planned suicide attempts.

Another group of narcissistic patients who may require inpatient or residential treatment are those with antisocial features. As described in Chapter 1, there is a continuum of narcissistic pathology that interfaces on the lower end with antisocial personality disorder. In tailoring treatment to these patients, one must make a careful assessment up front regarding whether the primary diagnosis is NPD associated with antisocial tendencies or true antisocial personality disorder (Gabbard 2014; Kernberg 2014). An essential aspect of this assessment is to acquire information from collateral sources because the patients themselves may consciously or unconsciously present a misleading or dishonest version of their history. *Some* patients with a pattern of deceptiveness and callousness toward others, that is, those with high motivation to change their behavior, may be treatable under carefully controlled conditions with intensive highly structured treatment. However, if the initial assessment determines that true antisocial personality disorder, or even malignant narcissism, is the diagnosis, any form of treatment is unlikely to succeed.

In patients with antisocial features, a residential setting that provides 24-hour observation is optimal but not always available because of the high cost of such treatment settings. In any case, the psychotherapist and the team involved in the treatment must have access to collateral sources so that the possibly deceptive account of a patient can be corroborated by external sources (Kernberg 2014). Much of the transference to the therapist is contaminated by deceptiveness and dishonesty such that outside information is absolutely essential for determining whether the therapist is being conned or being given accurate data. A structured setting is also ideal because of the risk for violence or criminal activity such as drug dealing or stealing. Patients in this category may also have comorbid substance abuse and may require detoxification followed by a rehabilitation program. A psychotherapeutically based treatment is unlikely to be effective until abstinence from substances has been achieved.

CONCLUSION

In this chapter we have elaborated a central theme that surfaces throughout the book: because of the pleomorphic nature of pathological narcissism, a generalization about one definitive approach is reductive and not clinically useful. We often stumble and grope in the dark a bit before discovering a strategy that is effective with the specific aspects of the patient's personality that causes distress to him or her and to others. This chapter's coverage of various treatments is by no means exhaustive.

REFERENCES

American Psychiatric Association: Diagnostic and Statistical Manual of Mental Disorders, 5th Edition. Arlington, VA, American Psychiatric Association, 2013

Bateman A, Fonagy P: Randomized controlled trial of outpatient mentalization-based treatment versus structured clinical management for borderline personality disorder. Am J Psychiatry 166(12):1355–1364, 2009 19833787

Bateman AW, Fonagy P (eds): Handbook of Mentalizing in Mental Health Practice. Arlington, VA, American Psychiatric Association, 2012

Bion WR: The Italian Seminars. Edited by Bion F, translated by Slotkin P. London, Karnac, 2005

Caligor E, Clarkin JF, Kernberg OF: Handbook of Dynamic Psychotherapy for Higher Level Personality Pathology. Washington, DC, American Psychiatric Publishing, 2007

Carsky M: Supportive psychoanalytic therapy for personality disorders. Psychotherapy (Chic) 50(3):443–448, 2013 24000868

Clarkin JF, Yeomans F, Kernberg OF: Psychotherapy of Borderline Personality: Focusing on Object Relations. Washington DC, American Psychiatric Publishing, 2006

Clarkin JF, Levy KN, Lenzenweger MF, et al: Evaluating three treatments for borderline personality disorder: a multiwave study. Am J Psychiatry 164(6):922–928, 2007 17541052

Connolly MB, Cris-Christoph P, Shappel S, et al: Relation of transference interpretations to outcome in early sessions of brief supportive-expressive psychotherapy. Psychother Res 9(4):485–495, 1999

Doering S, Hörz S, Rentrop M, et al: Transference-focused psychotherapy v. treatment by community psychotherapists for borderline personality disorder: randomised controlled trial. Br J Psychiatry 196(5):389–395, 2010 20435966

Doidge N, Simon B, Brauer L, et al: Psychoanalytic patients in the U.S., Canada, and Australia: I. DSM-III-R disorders, indications, previous treatment, medications, and length of treatment. J Am Psychoanal Assoc 50(2):575–614, 2002 12206544

Friedman L: What lies beyond interpretation, and is that the right question? Psychoanal Psychol 19:540–551, 2002

Gabbard GO: Psychodynamic Psychiatry in Clinical Practice, 5th Edition. Arlington, VA, American Psychiatric Publishing, 2014

Gabbard GO, Horwitz L, Allen JG, et al: Transference interpretation in the psychotherapy of borderline patients: a high-risk, high-gain phenomenon. Harv Rev Psychiatry 2(2):59–69, 1994 9384884

Gunderson JG, Hoffman ED (eds): Understanding and Treating Borderline Personality Disorder: A Guide for Professionals and Families. Arlington, VA, American Psychiatric Publishing, 2005

Høglend P, Gabbard GO: When is transference work useful in psychodynamic psychotherapy? A review of empirical research, in Handbook of Psychodynamic Psychotherapy: Evidence-Based Practice and Practice-Based Evidence. Edited by Levy RA, Ablon JS, Kächele H. New York, Humana Press, 2012, pp 449–470

Høglend P, Amlo S, Marble A, et al: Analysis of the patient-therapist relationship in dynamic psychotherapy: an experimental study of transference interpretations. Am J Psychiatry 163(10):1739–1746, 2006 17012684

Høglend P, Hersoug AG, Bøgwald KP, et al: Effects of transference work in the context of therapeutic alliance and quality of object relations. J Consult Clin Psychol 79(5):697–706, 2011 21859184

Kernberg OF: Borderline Conditions and Pathological Narcissism. New York, Jason Aronson, 1975

Kernberg OF: Severe Personality Disorders: Psychotherapeutic Strategies. New Haven, CT, Yale University Press, 1984

Kernberg OF: Narcissistic personality disorder, in Psychodynamic Psychotherapy for Personality Disorders: A Clinical Handbook. Edited by Clarkin JF, Fonagy P, Gabbard GO. Arlington, VA, American Psychiatric Publishing, 2010, pp 257–288

Kernberg OF: An overview of the treatment of severe narcissistic pathology. Int J Psychoanal 95(5): 865–888, 2014 24902768

Kohut H: The Analysis of the Self: A Systematic Approach to the Psychoanalytic Treatment of Narcissistic Personality Disorders. New York, International Universities Press, 1971

Kohut H: The Restoration of the Self. New York, International Universities Press, 1977

Levy KN, Meehan KB, Kelly KM, et al: Change in attachment patterns and reflective function in a randomized control trial of transference-focused psychotherapy for borderline personality disorder. J Consult Clin Psychol 74(6):1027–1040, 2006 17154733

Miller J: How Kohut actually worked. Progress in Self Psychology 1:13–30, 1985

Ogrodniczuk JS (ed): Understanding and Treating Pathological Narcissism. Washington, DC, American Psychological Association, 2013

Ogrodniczuk JS, Piper WE, Joyce AS, et al: Transference interpretations in short-term dynamic psychotherapy. J Nerv Ment Dis 187(9):571–578, 1999 10496513

Ogrodniczuk JS, Uliaszek AA, Lebow JL, Piper WE: Group, family, and couples therapies, in The American Psychiatric Publishing Textbook of Personality Disorders, 2nd Edition. Edited by Oldham JM, Skodol AE, Bender DS. Washington, DC, American Psychiatric Publishing, 2014, pp 281–302

Piper WE, Ogrodniczuk JS, Joyce AS, et al: Prediction of dropping out in time-limited, interpretative individual psychotherapy. Psychotherapy 36(2):114–122, 199, 1999

Ronningstam EF: Narcissistic personality disorder, in Gabbard's Treatments of Psychiatric Disorders, 5th Edition. Edited by Gabbard GO. Arlington, VA, American Psychiatric Publishing, 2014, pp 1073–1086

Stern BL, Yeomans F, Diamond D, et al: Transference-focused psychotherapy for narcissistic personality, in Understanding and Treating Pathological Narcissism. Edited by Agrodnozac JS. Washington, DC, American Psychological Association, 2013, pp 235–252

Wallerstein RW: Forty-Two Lives in Treatment: A Study of Psychoanalysis and Psychotherapy. New York, Guilford, 1986

Wong N: Clinical considerations in group treatment of narcissistic disorders. Int J Group Psychother 29(3):325–345, 1979 541142

7

Treatment Strategies

As the title of our book suggests, we are focusing our attention on common clinical dilemmas that come up in the treatment of narcissistic patients. Some of these have been noted in earlier chapters, where they were elaborated on and explained as being the outgrowth of narcissistic character pathology. In this chapter we elaborate on treatment ideas that were briefly touched on in Chapters 4–6. Specifically, we are going to provide selective strategies to deal with some of the most common and difficult challenges with narcissistic patients. We use the term *strategies* instead of *solutions* because some of these issues cannot be "solved." Rather, they have to be lived with and worked through as part of the treatment experience with narcissistically organized patients.

ENTITLEMENT, DEMANDS FOR SPECIAL TREATMENT, AND OMNIPOTENT CONTROL

As noted in Chapter 4, "Beginning the Treatment," the manner in which the patient presents is evident from the first phone call or meeting. With some narcissistic patients, the therapist is likely to be hijacked into a power struggle from the outset, whereas with others, the pressure can develop more gradually in the course of the treatment. This need to be in control persists throughout the treatment and does not occur only during the opening phases. One common dilemma is the following: to what extent does the therapist have to concede a degree of control to the patient in order to have a viable treatment? There is no definitive answer except to say that it falls under the category of clinical judgment. Patients may ask and even reasonably expect the therapist to modify in some manner what he or she does in order to meet the patient's needs, and with some patients these demands become untenable and over the top, an expression of the patient's sense of entitlement. Among the comments that a therapist is likely to hear are the following: "Since I am out of town during the week, can I see you Saturday?" "I have a payment coming that hasn't arrived yet, so I will just wait and pay you next month." "I had to cancel abruptly, and I can't believe you charged me for that." These expectations, questions, and demands of the therapist communicate the patient's belief that "I am an exception" and "The rules don't apply to me." Bion's (2005) notion that the patient is your best supervisor does not mean that the therapist's role should be construed as that of supervisee. Flexibility does not mean abdicating the therapeutic frame. Although the expectation for special treatment can and must be understood and discussed with a narcissistic patient in the therapy, it can also be a risk factor for descending the slippery slope to boundary violations (Gabbard 2016; Luchner 2013).

There is something strikingly irritating about the imperious style of some narcissistic patients, such that the therapist is tempted to convey an attitude of "my way or the highway." However, an important strategy is to continuously remind oneself that the patient's resistance reveals who he or she is. A basic premise in our work is that the patient is characterologically bound to do the therapy in the way he or she has to do it (Gabbard 2017). Moreover, because the patient's defenses become resistances when they appear in the treatment, the therapist is getting a glimpse of the characteristic defenses the patient uses against unbearable affect states.

As noted in Chapter 3, "Modes of Relatedness," research on narcissistic personality disorder (NPD) repeatedly identifies a pattern of omnipotent control as characteristic of the disorder. The patient has typically driven off many people in his or her life because he or she attempts to control them. The clinician strives to avoid being the next casualty. The therapist understands that he or she must partially submit to being controlled in order to have a viable treatment.

A helpful strategy in dealing with most of the narcissistic defenses, which become resistances when they enter the therapeutic relationship, is to remember that the resistances the patient is presenting tell the therapist who the patient is. In other words, resistance reveals as much as it conceals (Friedman 1991). This conceptualization fits nicely with what Roy Schafer (1983) referred to as an affirmative approach to resistance, one that focuses primarily on what resistance is for rather than on what it is against. In this affirmative approach, the therapist or analyst deemphasizes the notion that something is being resisted or opposed. Rather, the therapist examines the resistance as a puzzling or unintelligible behavior that cries out for understanding by the treater.

When the patient demands control over the treatment, the therapist is able to glimpse the deeply held fear in the narcissistic patient of the potential for others to hurt him or her if he or she relinquishes control (Gabbard 1998). Moreover, through the experience of being controlled by the patient, the therapist comes to feel controlled in much the same way as do others in the patient's life. Nevertheless, the clinician has to set limits according to what is manageable for him based on his background, his character structure, his theoretical models, and the structure of his clinical practice. In other words, a negotiation has to take place that grows out of the intersubjectivity of the dyad. The therapist needs to avoid the false polarity of giving in completely to the patient's demands or imposing overly strict limits.

The therapist is in a bind—if she wavers from her own treatment frame and acquiesces entirely to the patient's demands, she fosters the patient's sense that others are under his omnipotent control. On the other hand, if she draws a line in the sand and demands that the patient instead accommodate entirely to *her* omnipotent control, without budging at all, then she has only introjected the patient's controlling self and established a competitive showdown—that is, who is the boss? Neither pole is optimal. Instead, the clinician and patient must enter into a process. For example, if the patient demands an appointment time on Fridays at noon, the therapist should decline that possibility if the time is already filled. The therapist may find herself less willing than usual to look for alternatives, digging in her heels with the silent thought of "Who does he think he is?" Rather than give in to this more rigid manner of thinking that is growing out of her countertransference, she can reflect on this feeling of a showdown and offer a different option. Obviously, some of this processing of the countertransference may be easier between sessions. In the heat of the moment, one may be blinded to the best strategy by one's intense emotional reaction to the patient's demands. An ongoing mutual enactment will be played out as the treatment develops. This process is only the beginning. There is no "correct" answer, but it is enormously helpful to use a valued consultant who is not part of the dyad and can look at the power struggle from the outside.

> Mr. P, a 48-year-old executive, always arrived early for his appointments and sat in the waiting room with his electronic tablet, making a list of what to cover in the session. Dr. Q started each session with a hope that she would get a word in edgewise but knew her input was not welcome. She began to feel irritated and fantasized about coming to the session with her own list and giving her own monologue, when in fact, anytime she opened her mouth, she was always waved off and dismissed when Mr. P raised his hand and insisted, "just let me finish." Sometimes he gave her a raised hand or a shush without saying a word, continuing on as if she had not spoken. Without a doubt, Dr. Q's experience of being silenced by Mr. P was shaped by her own countertransference and her past experiences being silenced by someone in authority or being told her perspective was not important because of her gender.
>
> In her irritation at the many times Mr. P raised his hand to stop her from speaking, one day Dr. Q snapped, "You never want to hear my comments because you have to read your prepared monologue." He responded with consternation, saying, "I thought you would be so proud of me for bringing in all of this material for our work together! This is rich! You must be the only therapist alive who doesn't actually want me to plan what to talk about!" She replied, "I am glad you think about what we are doing outside of here, but I'm just trying to say I am not sure you feel that you want this to be a dialogue where we brainstorm together about what is going on." Mr. P retorted, "Well, no, that's not it. I just went to a lot of work to prepare all this stuff, and I feel you could at least let me finish before interrupting." Rather than digging further into a power struggle, Dr. Q took a deep breath and tried to recognize her own countertransferential contribution to their power struggle. They were both trying to be in the "one up" position and maintain control of the therapy, and neither of them wanted to budge. She asked him to go ahead with the list, thinking to herself to bring the issue up again at a time when both of them had cooler heads. She also made an appointment with a valued consultant to talk over what had transpired and how to conceptualize it.

The optimal strategy in this situation is probably to accommodate the patient's need to inform the therapist of his concerns. Some analysts and therapists have advocated telling the patient to turn off their electronic devices or to put down their lists. However, it is our belief that psychotherapy is not a coercive procedure. We allow patients to express themselves in the way they wish to, and we work with their need to have a prop, like a list on a tablet computer or smartphone, as something to be understood, not banished.

After tolerating a good deal of the patient's control in the service of forming a therapeutic alliance, the therapist may wish to bring up her dilemma with the patient, for example, "I don't mean to interrupt you, but I have trouble finding a space to offer my observations about what you're saying." In this way, the therapist engages the patient in a shared exploration of how her dilemma can be managed collaboratively. This inquiry opens up the possibility of discovering anxieties in the patient about being vulnerable. The therapist can wonder out loud about the nature of the patient's fear—is the patient concerned about what the therapist may think or say about him? Is the patient afraid of abdicating control if he allows the therapist to speak? Is he nervous about intimacy and being known by the therapist? In fact, the therapist *has* been quietly formulating hypotheses about the patient's modes of relatedness. The patient's fears are rooted in some sense of reality, that is, the therapist is thinking about the patient, and the patient may be most concerned about the possibility that the therapist will actually understand him. One of the most helpful things that a therapist can offer is an elucidation of the dialectic between exposure and concealment that is at the heart of the therapeutic dialogue.

In the example, Dr. Q made a decision to let go of the power struggle for now, planning to bring it up later when both the patient and therapist had cooler heads. Pine (1984) suggested that insight from the therapist is likely to be ignored when a patient is angry and agitated. He advised the therapist to instead "strike while the iron is cold" (p. 60). In our view, this strategy is useful with narcissistic patients, not only for the patient but also for the therapist. The therapist sometimes needs to wait until he or she has cooled down so as not to be interpreting through clenched teeth. An intervention is not only better received by the patient but often is more thoughtfully presented by the clinician when the heat of the iron has cooled.

BOREDOM, EXCLUSION, AND DISENGAGEMENT

As we noted in Chapter 5, "Transference and Countertransference" (see the section "Treating the Therapist Like a Sounding Board"), when treating a narcissistic patient, the therapist often feels as if the patient is talking to himself in the presence of the therapist. It feels as if the patient is talking not to the therapist specifically but rather to anyone within earshot. The therapist feels disengaged as the patient looks over her head, makes no eye contact, and drones on without expecting any interaction. A sense of dread fills the therapist before each session, and during the session, the clock seems to be frozen. Boredom can drift into sleepiness, which in turn can result in a narcissistic injury to the patient, who is understandably insulted by the therapist's lack of attention. The degree of aliveness versus deadness may be a useful barometer of how a treatment is going (Ogden 1995), and the lack of lively exchange between therapist and patient becomes unbearable to the therapist. In such situations, Ogden (1995) suggests that the analyst's strategy must be to create analytic meaning from that which has been present only unconsciously in the analytic dialogue and has been foreclosed from the analytic discourse.

It goes without saying that the patient has no obligation to entertain the clinician. It is the clinician's responsibility to maintain his or her own aliveness as well as to make boredom or disengagement a clinical problem. The clinician needs to use the countertransference in a way that moves the therapy forward. One cannot of course say to the patient that he is boring. Patrick Casement (1985) suggested a novel strategy involving a comment such as the following: "I have noticed, for some time now, that you frequently speak to me as if you are not expecting me to be interested in what you are saying" (pp. 169–170). Another variation that we have found effective is to say, "You don't sound terribly interested in what you are saying." In this way, the therapist is an active participant in the session rather than a passive victim of the deadening discourse.

Therapists must remember that their countertransference is taking them to meaningful places relevant to the therapeutic process. If the therapist starts to feel marginalized, irritated, or devalued, she can associate to her countertransference to detect any linkage to her own life or past, while also recognizing that she is probably feeling what others feel with the patient. Curiosity about the countertransference can keep the therapist's mind active and alive (Gabbard and Wilkinson 1994).

One way the therapist may be contributing to the boredom or disengagement is by repetitively interpreting patterns in the interaction. Many clinicians worry that the tradition of repeating and working through may not always lead to change. Brown and Elliott (2016) made the following assertion:

> We disagree with psychoanalytically oriented attachment-based treatments that primarily emphasize interpretation of reenactments of dysfunctional attachment behaviors in the transference relationship. Such

> treatments assume that insight about attachment patterns will lead to change in those patterns, but there is little evidence supporting such interpretation-based change. (p. 284)

Gabbard and Ogden (2009) have argued that some form of improvisation may be helpful for breaking out of the impasse. The "script" must be dropped at times, and the therapist must attempt to speak in a new mode, one that is unfamiliar to the patient. The therapist might, for example, say, "It seems to me that we've developed a pattern over time where I try to point out something you are doing, you disagree, and I go right on pointing it out anyway. Then we both feel frustrated. It's almost like we are colluding in frustrating each other."

SHAME, HUMILIATION, AND THE NECESSITY OF TACT

Narcissistic patients are often terribly self-critical and expect criticism and judgment from the therapist at every turn. The act of interpretation to clarify the projected experiences of self and other poses a major threat to the grandiose self of the patient (Steiner 2006; Stern et al. 2013). As noted in Chapter 1, "Narcissism and Its Discontents," narcissistically organized patients may have a fear of being seen by others for who they are. Hence, they gird themselves with psychological armor when they go into the battle of therapy. Interpretive understanding may appear to pierce that armor and leave the patient feeling exposed and humiliated. Hence, timing is of the utmost importance in the gradual confrontation of the grandiose self.

Patients may feel understood if the therapist focuses on the self-esteem struggles and insecurity underneath the surface, no matter how grandiose the façade seems to be. The fear of exposure and humiliation can be addressed empathically with the patient as a way of building up an alliance that will allow for interpretation of the grandiose aspects of the self. Some patients insist on pure empathy to fend off the shame, and therapists may feel that they have nothing left to give.

The therapist must constantly navigate a balance between empathy and confrontation/interpretation. Tact and timing are of great importance in monitoring the interventions of the therapist. In order to pave the way for interpretive comments, the therapist builds the alliance by noting the patient's successes and acknowledging his or her insight and progress. With some of the most sensitive and vigilant patients, clinicians can monitor how much they have compromised the patient's armor with an interpretive observation, watching the patient carefully to see how the insight is taken in. The best laid plans for interpretation are lost if they are met with immediate denial because the patient is too wounded and defensive to hear the interpretation or if the patient never returns.

When does the empathy become counterproductive? It is necessary to move beyond empathy with most narcissistic patients. In particular, when a patient has a tendency to look at the world through the lens of an aggrieved victim and to see every relationship and situation in this light, the therapist can point that out to the patient.

Kohut (1971, 1977) emphasized the difference between empathizing and agreeing with what the patient says, on the one hand, and empathizing with the pain and disappointment of not having one's needs for mirroring and validation met, on the other. There is a difference between taking the side of the patient and assuming his victimized perspective versus offering compassion about how much it must pain him that he did not get what he needed, either in childhood or in the here and now.

Narcissistic patients often brag about their accomplishments or name drop about famous people to whom they are connected. Therapists must tune in to the vulnerable self-esteem beneath the bragging in order to maintain a compassionate view of the patient that fosters the developing alliance. The focus on past successes—grade point averages, awards won, romantic conquests—can produce irritation in the therapist but also can be a place for the clinician to find the insecure child in the adult body of the patient. A therapist dealing with a patient who is boasting should be alert to the development of countertransference contempt, a wish to burst the patient's bubble or dismiss the cataloging of his or her victories and accomplishments. The therapist must contain that wish and recognize how important it is that the patient's accomplishments are witnessed by the therapist and how much the patient fears that people will not detect his or her special gifts.

RUPTURE AND REPAIR

Clinicians who attempt perfect empathy with their patients will always fail. A moment will inevitably emerge in which the therapist loses track of the conversation, tries to stifle a yawn, or behaves in an overt manner that shows a lack of empathy. Other, more subtle failures occur when a patient watches with hypervigilance for the therapist to be completely attuned, and the therapist misses it by a word or a sentence. The therapist's responsibility in this case is to move the treatment into a process of repair, reengagement, and exploring the patient's feelings about the empathic failure. Kohut's (1971, 1977) model of *rupture and repair* originated in one-person self psychology but has been appropriated by relational theory, intersubjectivity, and all other variants of two-person psychology. At this point in the evolution of the phrase, most therapists of all persuasions would agree that rupture and repair is a major mode of therapeutic action in psychotherapy and psychoanalysis.

Psychotherapy research supports this clinical observation. Stiles et al. (2004) found that alliance trajectories with brief, sharp declines and quick rebounds to original or higher levels predicted better outcomes of therapy. This finding suggested that temporary strains in the alliance are opportunities for deepening the therapeutic work. Safran et al. (2009) have defined the rupture-repair sequences with the alliance as problems in the therapeutic relationship that are repaired through interpersonal exploration between therapist and patient. This approach to disruptions in the alliance is useful in all therapies, but with narcissistic patients it is essential. Those who expect to be slighted and disrespected will find examples of therapist failures in virtually every session. The therapist needs to be open and nondefensive about the exploration of what the patient perceives and earnestly attempt to repair the breach. This model assists patients with NPD in understanding the two-way nature of ruptures. Both parties may contribute to the disruption, and both must be involved in negotiating the repair. In so doing, the narcissistically organized patient improves the capacity for mentalizing as well. This difficult moment in a therapeutic process is an opportunity for mutual recognition, as discussed in Chapter 5.

WHEN CHANGE IS NOT THE GOAL

Clinical experience teaches us that for a subgroup of narcissistic patients, change is not a realistic goal. Certain patients fall apart at *any* suggestion that they contribute to their own problems; hence, they may never be open to considering their role in the challenges they face, let alone trying to change how they relate to others in the world. In fact, it often seems that patients in this subgroup are not coming to therapy for change. They may come for various reasons, but secretly they hope that they will be validated and admired for who they are without the expectation that they need to change. In these patients, resistance is intransigent. Attempts to push for change or insight may lead to an abrupt and unilateral termination. A further complication is that these patients are not easily identified at the outset of treatment. Only through repeated failures to engage them in an active reflective process, one where all attempts at interpretation or confrontation are met with anger, denial, or distance, does the therapist get the full picture. The therapist must come to the reluctant conclusion that the patient simply cannot tolerate anything beyond empathy, support, and agreement.

This form of impasse is widely experienced by practitioners but is perhaps underreported in the literature. Some therapists may assume it is *their* failure, rather than a fundamental limitation of the patient, and therefore wish to keep their experience to themselves. In our experience, this scenario is not uncommon, and clinicians find ways to work within the limits. In such a situation, the clinician must lower expectations about what is possible in the therapy. The therapist's shift in expectations is often followed by a sense of relief in the patient, who may have felt that she simply was failing to do the therapy "correctly." It is difficult for the therapist to ask himself, "What am I doing here if nothing is really changing and I don't challenge her or point out things that get in her way?" In addition to witnessing and trying sincerely to understand the patient's story, the therapist is providing a place for the patient to vent her hurts and disappointments. Perhaps the therapist is also taking some of the burden off of family members, who can develop empathy fatigue and may erupt in irritation.

Clinicians should keep in mind that there are some patients who tend to look at the world as a series of narcissistic slights and injuries and who *must* have a bad object in their lives. Treatment may threaten them with the loss of that necessary tormenter. Therapists and analysts who are struggling with a tenacious patient who insists on a victim narrative are advised to remember the material in Chapter 5 regarding the narcissistic-masochistic character (Cooper 1993, 2009). A form of specialness is extracted by the perception that the treater is repeatedly failing the patient or slighting him or her in some way. The patient is seeking in the outer world the "bad-enough object" who resides in his or her inner world.

Of course, most therapists would try to help patients see how they create "bad objects" in their lives and would challenge that expectation, hoping to change the entrenched view. However, we wish to emphasize that for some narcissistically organized patients, this ability is not within reach. One strategy in these situations is to shift the expectation from insight and change and instead ally with the patient in an effort to keep the tormenting object affixed to a less important person, group, or institution. In other words, part of the supportive therapy process here is to avoid interfering with the displacement of the bad object onto a figure other than spouse, partner, or boss. Grievance collectors must have their grievances, and therapists need to respect that. An ongoing feud with the dry cleaner may be far better than an ongoing attack on one's spouse or child. The therapist who tolerates lengthy rants about a political party may be deflecting the patient's discontent with his or her boss.

Another strategy is to try to help the patient see the downside of getting into confrontations—leaving a voice mail with a barrage of angry and entitled rants for a boss or friend, for example, does not usually end well. The therapist maintains a strategy of trying to empathize with the patient and hear how awful he feels, all the while trying to get him to slow down and not leave such angry voice mails by seeing the potential consequences of his rage. These strategies do not work toward fundamental character change but rather may be small shifts in behavior that one hopes will make a sustained impact on the patient's overall well-being in relationships and work settings. With this strategy, one may observe the paradox that the patient has not changed but is "better." Therapists would be well advised to consider Winnicott's (1971) wise comment: "Psychotherapy is not making clever and apt interpretation; by and large it is a long-term giving back to the patient what the patient brings. It is a complex derivative of the face that reflects what is there to be seen" (p. 158).

IDEALIZATION

Idealization of the other leading to an enhanced view of the self by being in the shadow of the idealized object is one way that narcissistic patients sustain their self-esteem (Kohut 1971, 1977). Some idealization of the therapist can be helpful for the therapeutic alliance, and initially, it may certainly feel more pleasant to the therapist than a hostile transference. However, continued overt idealization can be uncomfortable for the therapist and detrimental to the treatment. In addition, idealization will sooner or later crumble and therefore is unlikely to serve as a solid foundation for the treatment relationship over the long term.

It is possible to maintain a positive transference unless it is causing problems, but there is a risk that too much idealization can lead to the tendency to develop a "mutual admiration society" between patient and therapist. As the patient basks in the glow of the idealized therapist's bright reflection, the patient showers the therapist with compliments. Feeling that his or her own narcissistic needs are being gratified, the therapist may feel tempted to return the compliments and begins to see the patient in an overly positive light. As the glowing reflections are passed back and forth between them, the danger is that the real work of the therapy is lost. The therapist colludes with the patient in avoiding the negative aspects of the patient's life while also steering clear of the self-scrutiny that is inherent in the therapeutic endeavor (Gabbard 1998, 2013).

When the therapist feels idealized in this way, he or she can leave the transference alone for a while and let it unfold, while also predicting that at some point he or she will undoubtedly disappoint the patient. Sometimes, one can approach this mutual admiration society with a sense of humor, chuckling a bit at one's "sainthood," and then try to redirect the patient to his or her own problems. If the idealization becomes rigidly fixed, a more active exploration can be indicated. The therapist can help the patient look at what he or she is defending against in trying to keep the relationship idealized. Fears of criticism, abandonment, or loss of control can sometimes underlie idealization and a wish to please the therapist.

ENVY AND COMPETITIVENESS

Envy of the therapist is a major force responsible for failed treatments. For the narcissistic patient, "there can only be one great person in the room" (Kernberg 2010, p. 266). The narcissistic patient often feels he or she is trapped in a one-down position, when he or she instead wants to be the one in control. As noted in Chapter 6, "Tailoring the Treatment to the Patient," in the patient's mind, a dichotomy exists in which one person is always superior and the other is devalued, demeaned, or ignored (Stern et al. 2013). In this dyad, either the patient experiences himself or herself as the devalued one and the therapist as the vaunted and superior other, or the situation is reversed and the patient is in the superior position while the therapist is devalued. This dichotomy is at the heart of transference-focused psychotherapy. In the process of the ongoing working through with these patients, the therapist interprets the roles that each is taking in the dyad, as described in Chapter 6.

These patients feel despair at someone else's success and feel joy when someone else fails. Envy causes them to link themselves directly with others they view as competitors. There is not enough of the pie to go around—if someone else gets a piece, they will get less. In the zero-sum game of envy, there is a myth that if someone has something good, the other person is diminished. A major goal of therapy is to help patients see that self-esteem is not dependent on what someone else has and that their accomplishments are not connected to those of others. The therapist works to interpret to the patient that his zero-sum view undermines the chance in his life that he and others can simultaneously feel successful and gratified. A major thrust of the treatment is to convince the patient that there is actually enough room for two people to be successful in the same endeavor. This is a core theme in narcissistic individuals, and the dynamics of comparison and envy are further mediated by the culture, as the expansion of social media fans the flames of competitiveness and insecurity (see Chapter 2, "The Cultural Context of Narcissism"). Glamorous photos of a person's incomparable life disseminated to hundreds of "friends" can certainly contribute to a feeling of how much is missing from one's own life.

THE CONTEMPTUOUS PATIENT

With the contemptuous patient, a barrage of criticism takes its toll on the therapist's capacity to think. The therapist feels narcissistically wounded, devalued, and deskilled. He or she feels robbed of the ability to feel helpful and gratified (Gabbard 2000). With these patients, the clinician must be aware of the development of countertransference contempt in return, which might lead to an enactment in which the therapist returns fire with fire. The therapist must tolerate some degree of contempt, but only up to a point. When contempt cuts too deep, the therapist must be able to set limits. The exact point at which the limits are implemented differs from one therapist to another. The therapist must find a way to maintain his or her own reflective capacity in the face of criticism, as the tendency is to retreat into "fight versus flight" and either say nothing or engage the patient in a contemptuous face-off. Supervision or consultation can help the therapist to contain and metabolize some of the demeaning comments so that he or she can continue to function as the therapist and think his or her own thoughts (Gabbard and Wilkinson 1994). As the therapist tries to process his or her own experience, he or she can also attempt to connect with the patient's feelings underneath the barrage of criticism by tuning in to the patient's fears and insecurities. Underneath all the bullying bravado is often a desperately insecure person.

> Mr. R spent several sessions berating Dr. S with a series of humbling and nasty comments. "I cannot believe you just said that—what a stupid thing to say! Really! Is that all you've got? Isn't there anything in all those books on the shelf that you could say that could be a tiny bit helpful to me? Do I need to read them to you? Maybe I can assign you homework—go home and actually read something about how to do psychiatry! Didn't they teach you anything in residency? I thought my last three therapists were bad, but then I met you!" Dr. S found herself

shrinking back in her chair, becoming quieter and quieter, saying less and less each subsequent session. Once she realized she was unconsciously trying to avoid the tirade and that Mr. R's criticism made her feel less secure in her ability to help him as a therapist, she sought consultation.

In moments when the therapist cannot think during the session, often the best course of action is to do some self-reflection and seek consultation and return to the therapy with the advice of the consultant in mind, with more of a "plan" about how to proceed. Dr. S did so, and the next time the barrage started, she said, "I know you are unhappy about what I am doing—you have been pretty critical of me. Can we talk about what's going on? Are you afraid that I'm not good enough to help you?"

Another strategy is to work within the transference to grasp what is being repeated from the past. Is this a reenactment of a bully-victim dynamic from the patient's past—perhaps as a child he was shamed by a critical parent? Could it be that the recapitulation of that experience over time with the therapist (and others) is an attempt at active mastery over passively experienced trauma?

THE PATIENT WHO CAN'T (OR WON'T) MENTALIZE

As discussed in Chapter 3, a common problem in narcissistic patients is that the patient is unable to imagine the perspective of the other. In these patients, much of the therapeutic work is in the back and forth of the therapist's teaching and modeling of mentalizing (Bateman and Fonagy 2012). Comments from the therapist's perspective, such as "What did you imagine I was thinking?" or "Were you worried about how I would react?" or "I can imagine feeling sad and angry about that if I had been in that situation," are some of the fundamentals of teaching this skill to patients. A psychoeducational approach may be less likely to wound the patient than would a confrontation about his or her self-centeredness. These comments may be about mentalizing what is going on in the mind of the therapist or asking the patient to imagine the inner world of the patient's family and people in his or her life. In concrete examples, even role-played at times, the therapist may ask questions such as "How do you think your wife felt when you left without saying goodbye?" or "How did you imagine your boss perceived you after you told him that you wouldn't take on the project he asked you to do because it wasn't your job?" or "What do you think your son felt when you yelled and slammed the door?"

There are other patients who *can* mentalize but simply do not care what the other person thinks or feels.

> Mr. T, a 63-year-old CEO, complained about sitting in a meeting with his board of directors: "I am so sick and tired of listening to all the different opinions in the room. I don't really give a damn what any of them think. I know what to do, but I have to put up a pretense of interest in their comments."

This attitude toward the contributions of others can be a challenge for the therapist who is trying to encourage the patient to appreciate the value of mentalizing. Often, a patient who becomes focused on being "right" or "in charge" needs help in seeing the value of taking others' perspectives into account. Oblivious patients may require a "2 by 4 approach" in which the therapist makes a bold confrontation to gain the patient's attention—symbolically "bopping" the patient on the head. The therapist might say, for example, "I don't think you heard a word of what I just said to you." However, this same manner of interpretation would be too harsh for a more hypervigilant patient.

NARCISSISTIC RAGE

Patients who explode with rage at being hurt, misunderstood, or slighted pose a particular problem in the consulting room. The patient feels terrified that he is not being heard or honored, and his rage covers over his fear and disappointment in the therapist. When a patient behaves explosively, the therapist may feel frightened and panicky. First and foremost, the clinician must feel safe to do his or her job. As Harold Searles (personal communication, January 1993) once quipped, "The therapist's chair must be more comfortable than the patient's chair." The patient's narcissism may be accompanied by a form of pathological certainty that is intimidating to the therapist, who may wonder to herself, "Maybe I did make a stupid comment!" Moreover, a patient who is screaming at the therapist may cause the therapist to freeze. The atmosphere created by a raging patient is not conducive to thought. The best the therapist may be able to do is sit, contain, and take a few deep breaths. The therapist may also need to say, "I find it impossible to think when you are screaming at me."

When the dust settles—either in the same session or later—the therapist may feel more capable of processing what happened with the patient. Containing the rage-fueled transference as well as one's own countertransference is a high expectation, and no therapist can completely master this form of holding. The therapist herself may feel caught and ashamed when her patient is raging at her. Another disconcerting development is when the rage in the patient provokes a feeling of rage in the therapist, and the therapist must make an effort to calm down and deescalate the anger of both participants. Some therapists may also feel a knee-jerk reaction of contempt or ridicule toward the patient. Scorn, dismissiveness, or nervous laughter in disbelief may occur in the face of a patient's over-the-top, unnecessary explosion following a relatively minor slight.

Virtually every interaction between patient and therapist is intersubjective, and moments of anger and rage can certainly be co-constructed and bidirectional. Enactments that lead to firing patients, leaving sessions, and having feelings of righteous indignation or justification can be countertransference responses that lead to rupture without repair. Consultation with a colleague after a session filled with rage may help guide one through this countertransference tempest.

CHARM AS A DEFENSE

With patients in the high-functioning subtype, a major challenge for the therapist may be to avoid being blinded by the glaring charm of the patient in order to engage in a deeper way that sees through the surface presentation. Although these patients are charming and interesting and appear to be motivated for therapy, over time the therapist comes to see that the appearance of engagement in therapy is a version of Winnicott's (1965) false self adaptation designed to win over the therapist as they have won over others in their lives.

In the countertransference with Mrs. K described in Chapter 5, Dr. L discovers that the superficial manner in which Mrs. K participates in therapy is aimed at pleasing the therapist rather than garnering insight about herself. Dr. L starts to realize that Mrs. K does not make connections between sessions and feels himself becoming disengaged. This awareness is where the work begins. Certainly, Dr. L must look at his countertransference detachment as a marker for how others in Mrs. K's life experience her. Rather than letting the detachment happen, Dr. L now has the chance to share with Mrs. K his experience of her and talk about seeking to understand her underlying anxieties.

Because high-functioning patients are not as brittle as those in the other narcissistic subtypes, Dr. L might introduce the point that he finds that each session starts anew, that "we don't often pick up the thread of our conversation from last time—and I wonder what you have been thinking and feeling about what we have discussed." High-functioning narcissists are prone to shame and may be quite attuned to pleasing the therapist, so the therapist must always be aware of the need for balance between making a helpful observation, on the one hand, and speaking in a way that shames the patient, on the other. As the therapist works to keep himself or herself engaged and active in a treatment that feels alive, he or she attempts to draw the patient more deeply into a genuine process of therapy, and of life, rather than engaging in a superficial process.

SUICIDALITY

The literature on suicide risk tends to emphasize that suicidal feelings grow out of preexisting mood disorders and/or substance abuse. There is far less emphasis on the fact that an acute narcissistic injury can produce intense shame and humiliation to the point where suicide seems like the only option available. In such situations, a narcissistically organized person can feel that he or she has been shattered forever and that no form of redemption is possible. This utter hopelessness can lead to a feeling best described as "my life is over." Hence, suicide may become thinkable for the first time in someone who has had a long string of successes. Links (2013) emphasized that in a narcissistically disturbed person, the wish to kill oneself can emerge without the presence of a depressed state. That wish can emerge from a desperate need to regulate self-esteem or to protect a pathological self-image. Inpatient hospitalization may be essential to prevent a tragedy. Kernberg (2010) stressed that acute suicide risk connected with narcissistic injury must be differentiated from the chronically suicidal patient who has used suicidal threats to manipulate others.

Chronically suicidal patients can sometimes be treated as an outpatient provided that the patient can assure his or her safety to the therapist. The state of the therapeutic alliance is highly significant in determining whether an inpatient stay is needed. Because narcissistic patients may form superficial pseudo alliances with their therapists, a thoroughgoing discussion with suicidal patients about their capacity to communicate is essential. Where there is a solid alliance, outpatient therapy may provide a setting to examine the triggers for the suicidality; the fantasies of what suicide will accomplish; and the consequences to others, such as family members, if the suicide is completed.

The patient may simultaneously long for the therapist to be a godlike figure who will save him or her while also wishing to destroy the therapist and ruin the therapist's reputation (Kernberg 2014). Narcissistic patients may disparage the therapist's competence by accusing him or her of being inattentive or oblivious to their lethality. At the same time, they may expect their therapist to know what they are thinking without having to say it. Therapists in such situations must explain that they cannot read minds and that only a collaborative effort between patient and therapist can get to the root of the feeling that suicide is the only way out.

There is a difference between treatment and management of the suicidal patient (Gabbard 2014). *Management* involves removing sharp objects from the patient's environment, continuous observation in a hospital, and sometimes even restraints. These measures do not necessarily decrease the patient's future vulnerability to suicide. *Treatment*, on the other hand, is geared toward altering the wish to die. It involves a therapeutic effort to discover the patient's fantasies associated with suicide and the evolution of the self-loathing that led to the decision to take one's life. Psychotherapy focusing on internal factors and external stressors and, when indicated, prescription of medication are the major tools of treatment.

The relentlessly suicidal patient with narcissistic features may take pleasure in tormenting the therapist. Maltsberger and Buie (1974) noted that feelings of malice and aversion are among the most common countertransference reactions connected with the treatment of severely suicidal patients. Clinicians involved with the treatment may find it extraordinarily challenging to tolerate their own sadistic wishes toward a patient who is tormenting them with contempt toward the therapist and a refusal to collaborate in treatment. These wishes may lead to an aversion on the clinicians' part to their involvement, unconsciously contributing to a suicide attempt.

A subgroup of narcissistic patients may voice suicidal thoughts when they feel the therapist has not been attuned to their needs or has chosen not to gratify their requests for extended sessions, numerous phone calls, and meetings outside the office. The narcissist with masochistic characteristics may complain vociferously about the therapist's shortcomings and how the therapist is "driving me to suicide." These patients may feel entitled to round-the-clock contact with the therapist and feel terribly victimized when it is not granted. They may fantasize that they will go out in a "blaze of glory" to destroy the therapist. The patient dangles the threat of suicide over his or her own head like the sword of Damocles, and the therapist is likely to respond with countertransference hatred. Therapists must repeatedly strive to distinguish between what is the therapist's responsibility and what is the patient's responsibility. Finally, as clinicians, we must acknowledge the limits of what is possible—in the final analysis, we cannot stop someone from killing himself or herself. That decision will ultimately be the patient's.

THE AGING NARCISSIST

In a study of 262 undergraduates, Rose (2002) found that individuals who fit the profile of the grandiose or overt narcissist may rate themselves high on measures of happiness and self-esteem. One can infer that they may actually derive certain psychological benefits from self-deception that ordinary people do not enjoy. By regarding others as inferior and maintaining unrealistic beliefs about themselves, they can defend against pain and shame. Some may have notable successes in work and love as young adults. However, the ravages of aging and the inalterable certainty of death may lead to intense suffering. Some deny the frailties of the body by taking up marathon running or sexual promiscuity. Others undergo religious conversions. One of the tragedies facing narcissistic individuals is that they have great difficulty in deriving vicarious pleasure from the successes of their children or mentees because of their envy and despair. They may find themselves isolated and thus seek psychotherapy for the first time in their lives.

The crisis of aging and the confrontation with mortality is an opportunity for the clinician as well. Whereas some thrust themselves into activities driven by manic defenses, others become capable of mourning and recognizing the folly of pursuing perfection. The body will never again look like it did at the age of 25. The dream of a Nobel Prize will never come to fruition. When one reaches one's 60s and 70s, retirement and death must be faced. As noted in Chapter 1, a tragic aspect of pathological perfectionism is that the pursuit of the Holy Grail (in whatever form it may take for each individual) prevents one from living in the moment and taking pleasure in the ebb and flow of daily living. Part of the mourning process is to deal with the sobering realization that one has missed one's life to some extent.

> Dr. U, a 71-year-old academic, retired from his position at a university, knowing that he had a form of bone cancer that was not responsive to radiation or chemotherapy. He came to a therapist for the first time. His opening statement was "I'm becoming irrelevant." He went on to say that his whole self-esteem was based on his academic achievements. His position had now been taken away from him, and he did not know what to do. No one would be following his publications and valuing his work anymore. In one session after another, Dr. U expressed self-loathing for how he had lived his life. He confided that he never felt that he really lived up to his potential even though he was a highly respected figure in

his field. The therapist asked what his regrets were. Dr. U took a deep breath, paused, and then replied that he had always neglected his wife and his children. He felt that he had been callous to the needs of his family and had irreparably damaged them. The therapist pointed out that there was still time to do something about that. Dr. U started to tear up. He told his therapist that his wife and children had such bitterness that they would never forgive him. His sense of shame was overwhelming. The therapist stressed that Dr. U was not "irrelevant" to his family and encouraged him to make an effort to connect in some way while the clock was still ticking. For the first time, Dr. U was able to acknowledge the harm he had done to his family and apologize to them.

Death is the ultimate narcissistic injury. Some people seek to find a way around it. Others face it with panic and rage. Therapists can help patients focus on their mortality. The approach of death presents an opportunity to make peace with those whom one has neglected, as with Dr. U. Moreover, it offers the patient a chance to reflect on what one has accomplished, where one has failed, and to recognize that perfection is unattainable. The goal of such work is to come to a more balanced and nuanced understanding of one's achievements and failures.

CONCLUSION

This collection of treatment strategies is incomplete by necessity. Every treatment has idiosyncratic qualities that cannot be easily generalized. We have assembled what we consider to be a few of the highly prevalent clinical experiences in working with narcissistic patients. In many situations, the therapist relies on improvisation and thinking in the moment because unexpected developments are virtually universal in the treatment of narcissistic patients.

REFERENCES

Bateman A, Fonagy P: Handbook of Mentalizing in Mental Health Practice. Arlington, VA, American Psychiatric Publishing, 2012
Bion WR: The Italian Seminars. Edited by Bion F, translated by Slotkin P. London, Karnac, 2005
Brown DP, Elliott DS: Attachment Disturbances in Adults: Treatment for Comprehensive Repair. New York, WW Norton, 2016
Casement P: Further Learning From the Patient. London, Tavistock, 1985
Cooper AM: Psychotherapeutic approaches to masochism. J Psychother Pract Res 2(1):51–63, 1993 22700126
Cooper AM: The narcissistic-masochistic character. Psychiatr Ann 39:904–912, 2009

Friedman L: A reading of Freud's papers on technique. Psychoanal Q 60(4):564–595, 1991 1758912

Gabbard GO: Transference and countertransference in the treatment of narcissistic patients, in Disorders of Narcissism: Diagnostic, Clinical and Empirical Implications. Edited by Ronningstam EF. Washington, DC, American Psychiatric Press, 1998, pp 125–146

Gabbard GO: On gratitude and gratification. J Am Psychoanal Assoc 48(3):697–716, 2000 11059393

Gabbard GO: Countertransference issues in the treatment of pathological narcissism, in Understanding and Treating Pathological Narcissism. Edited by Ogrodniczuk JS. Washington DC, American Psychological Association, 2013, pp 207–217

Gabbard GO: Psychodynamic Psychiatry in Clinical Practice, 5th Edition. Arlington, VA, American Psychiatric Publishing, 2014

Gabbard GO: Boundaries and Boundary Violations, 2nd Edition. Arlington, VA, American Psychiatric Association Publishing, 2016

Gabbard GO: Long-Term Psychodynamic Psychotherapy: A Basic Text, 3rd Edition. Arlington, VA, American Psychiatric Association Publishing, 2017

Gabbard GO, Wilkinson SM: Management of Countertransference With Borderline Patients. Washington, DC, American Psychiatric Press, 1994

Gabbard GO, Ogden TH: On becoming a psychoanalyst. Int J Psychoanal 90(2):311–327, 2009 19382962

Kernberg OF: Narcissistic personality disorder, in Psychodynamic Psychotherapy for Personality Disorders: A Clinical Handbook. Edited by Clarkin JF, Fonagy P, Gabbard GO. Washington, DC, American Psychiatric Publishing, 2010, pp. 257–287

Kernberg OF: An overview of the treatment of severe narcissistic pathology. Int J Psychoanal 95(5):865–888, 2014 24902768

Kohut H: The Analysis of the Self: A Systematic Approach to the Psychoanalytic Treatment of Narcissistic Personality Disorders. New York, International Universities Press, 1971

Kohut H: The Restoration of the Self. New York, International Universities Press, 1977

Links PS: Pathological narcissism and the risk of suicide, in Understanding and Treating Pathological Narcissism. Edited by Ogrodniczuk JS. Washington, DC, American Psychological Association, 2013, pp 167–182

Luchner AF: Maintaining boundaries in the treatment of pathological narcissism, in Understanding and Treating Pathological Narcissism. Edited by Ogrodniczuk JS. Washington DC, American Psychological Association, 2013, pp 219–234

Maltsberger JT, Buie DH: Countertransference hate in the treatment of suicidal patients. Arch Gen Psychiatry 30(5):625–633, 1974 4824197

Ogden TH: Analysing forms of aliveness and deadness of the transference-countertransference. Int J Psychoanal 76(Pt 4):695–709, 1995 8543428

Pine F: The interpretive moment: variations on classical themes. Bull Menninger Clin 48(1):54–71, 1984 6692050

Rose P: The happy and unhappy faces of narcissism. Pers Individ Dif 33:379–391, 2002

Safran J, Muran JC, Proskurov B: Alliance, negotiation, and rupture resolution, in Handbook of Evidence-Based Psychodynamic Psychotherapy. Edited by Levy RA, Ablon JS. New York, Humana Press, 2009, pp 201–255

Schafer R: The Analytic Attitude. New York, Basic Books, 1983

Steiner J: Seeing and being seen: narcissistic pride and narcissistic humiliation. Int J Psychoanal 87(Pt 4):939–951, 2006 16877245

Stern BL, Yeomans F, Diamond D, et al: Transference-focused psychotherapy for narcissistic personality, in Understanding and Treating Pathological Narcissism. Edited by Ogrodniczuk JS. Washington, DC, American Psychological Association, 2013, pp 235–252

Stiles WB, Glick MJ, Osatuke K, et al: Patterns of alliance development and the rupture-repair hypothesis; are productive relationships U-shaped or V-shaped? J Couns Psychol 51(1):81–92, 2004

Winnicott DW: Ego distortion in terms of true and false self (1960), in The Maturational Processes and the Facilitating Environment. New York, International Universities Press, 1965, pp 140–152

Winnicott DW: Playing and Reality. London, Penguin, 1971

8

Termination

The psychoanalytic literature on termination of treatment is fraught with myths and mythologizing (Gabbard 2009; Kantrowitz 2015). Part of the long-standing mythology is that the patient comes to analysis with a set of problems and struggles to understand them, and the analyst deftly analyzes the core conflicts, especially as they emerge in the transference. The patient feels grateful and undergoes an orderly termination process of a few months and then embarks on a new life thanks to the analyst and the analytic process. However, Judy Kantrowitz (2015) systematically conducted interviews of 82 former analytic patients and found that analysis terminates in many different ways such that a "standard approach" to termination would be highly misleading. There can be little doubt that termination has been idealized in much of psychoanalytic writing. The common experience of psychoanalytic candidates is a growing awareness that their control cases do not adhere to the model of termination that they were taught. Like much of life experience outside of treatment, termination is often messy.

The focus of psychoanalytic treatments, whether psychoanalysis proper or psychoanalytic therapy, is that which is unique, idiosyncratic, and specific to the patient (Gabbard 2007). Hence, the termination of any one particular patient by one particular analyst does not lend itself to reductive formulations or technical approaches. The literature of classical psychoanalysis is replete with idealized expectations regarding a good termination: the modification of the superego, the ability to love and work, the eradication of symptoms, the achievement of "full genitality," and the interpretive resolution of the transference neurosis. Freud (1937/1955) actually viewed termination as "a practical matter" (p. 249). He stressed that unpredictable developments in the course of the treatment—for example, financial setbacks, relocation—would arise and play a major role in how analysis ends. The practical was emphasized in contrast to the ideal.

TERMINATION OF NARCISSISTIC PATIENTS

If we turn from the *general* topic of termination to the *specific* problems encountered in the termination of narcissistic patients, we discover formidable challenges. Brunell and Campbell (2011) pointed out that many narcissists actually feel good about themselves and thus may not be interested in changing anything. They may have a perspective that they are superior to others and see no compelling reason to change how they are. A series of failures may be necessary to bring them into treatment, but they may wish to terminate long before substantive change occurs.

Kernberg (1975) has acknowledged that the overall prognosis for persons with narcissistic personality disorder (NPD) is guarded. Although narcissistic patients often appear to be in the center of events, they function within a psychological shell of isolation that may insulate them from meaningful emotional relationships and from the potential for narcissistic wounds. A set of narcissistic resistances arises from the patient's incapacity to depend on another person (Kernberg et al. 1989). As noted in Chapter 7," Specific Treatment Strategies," omnipotent control is present in the vast majority of patients with narcissistic difficulties despite their level of functioning, and this need to control the treatment may be a pervasive resistance to receiving help. Kernberg (2014) notes that these patients unconsciously "freeze" the therapeutic situation and thus protect their grandiose self from any form of modification. They tend to lack trust in the therapist as someone who is genuinely interested in them. They may refuse to accept the therapist's observations and interpretations, stating that they already know what the therapist is trying to explain. Moreover, envy of the therapist is a prominent issue in the treatment, and these patients need to spoil any ideas of the therapist to avoid being taken over by even more intense envy.

The prognosis for such patients may improve a bit if there is some capacity for depression and mourning. Those with a degree of superego integration are likely to have a better prognosis as well. Narcissistically organized patients may conceptualize the goals of therapy as a means to enhance their positive qualities. One young professional told his therapist in the first session that his major goal in seeking treatment was to become "even more perfect." If such a patient has been able to use the therapy to question his perfectionism, reflect on it, and open his eyes to a more realistic set of expectations, his treatment may come to a more satisfactory conclusion than that of a patient who is truly unwilling to relinquish an unattainable goal. Moreover, a patient's pressure for the clinician to constantly admire his "perfection," rather than pointing out areas that might need some work, can set up a stalemate in the psychotherapeutic process that may not end well.

Narcissistic patients may take years of treatment before changes are apparent that might cause the therapist or analyst to begin to think about termination. The patients may grow to tolerate envy a little bit better, and they may develop a sense of guilt about having hurt others or the therapist. Kernberg (1975) noted that a good prognostic sign is when their envy can be transformed into jealousy within a triangular relationship. A reliable predictor of poor outcome, of course, is the presence of severe antisocial tendencies.

As discussed in Chapter 1, "Narcissism and Its Discontents," narcissistic struggles occur on a continuum, and patients who have narcissistic tendencies, rather than NPD proper, are often able to make significant gains in psychotherapy or psychoanalysis. Therapists are able to make some progress with patients who gain skills in mentalizing the perspectives of their loved ones and colleagues. Focusing on perfectionism, with the reminder that "the perfect is the enemy of the good," may help patients develop more realistic expectations of life as well as mourn unmet fantasies of how their lives and careers should have been "the best." Termination may be a natural result of a therapeutic process in which a patient has been able to decrease her constant comparisons of herself to others and work through her envy. As she does so, she gains the ability to imagine that a zero-sum game is not actually how the world works, and hence she can increasingly appreciate and celebrate the successes of others without fearing that her own specialness is in jeopardy.

> Ms. V, a young woman in her early 30s, felt "tortured" by her sense that others always have what she wants and she is always left in the lurch. She watched her friends on social media, posting great successes and happy pictures of their love lives while looking fabulous and seeming like they have "perfect" lives. She dropped one relationship after another when the "fabulous" man of the moment turned out to be yet another example of "just your average disappointment." She started the therapy with an unrealistic goal: "I want to be on cloud nine like everyone else. All of my friends have better relationships than I do. Everyone else has it all together. It's not fair." As she was able to gradually realize that most social media posts are cultivated and do not represent the whole picture of anyone's life, she began to imagine that her friends have struggles just as she does in her relationships. With repeated efforts at empathy and interpretation on the part of the therapist, she said, "After all this time in therapy, I still feel envious sometimes when I see my friends, but now I am more able to embrace the fact that no one actually has it a lot better than I do. Well, maybe some people truly do, but most are pretty much in the same place as me." She said that she felt less plagued by the constant envious comparisons and could see that all relationships are imbued with ambivalence. Her recognition that some disappointment is inevitable became the foundation for a successful termination in which she could leave therapy and approach her life and relationships with more realistic expectations and feel less tormented by constant envious comparisons. She has been more able to accept the mundane pleasures in her life without expecting every moment to be "cloud nine."

Systematic consideration of termination with NPD patients has been greatly hampered by the fact that sudden dropouts and premature termination are pervasive within this population of patients (Ronningstam 2014). Many patients are overwhelmed by their sense of vulnerability in treatment and develop a paranoid orientation to the process that may lead them to flee. In addition, a treatment that is trying to help the patient integrate aspects of self and other can be viewed by the patient as destabilizing, leading to sudden disappearances from appointments without explanation. Finally, the illusion of perfection will also be threatened when the patient's insecurities, misperceptions, or self-doubts are pointed out.

The countertransferences described in Chapter 5, "Transference and Countertransference," may also contribute to premature termination. The therapist or analyst who treats a narcissistic patient is likely to suffer the slings and arrows of outrageous transference. Contempt, devaluation, and sarcastic mockery of all attempts to provide understanding may be a daily experience. Therapists may be driven to respond, as noted in Chapter 5, by engaging in an enactment in which they retaliate by being overtly confrontational or by using interpretations as attacks, thus confirming the critical opinion of the patient.

> Mr. W had been in psychotherapy for 2 months and grew increasingly impatient with the therapist, Dr. X.
>
> > **Mr. W:** I'm not sure this process is worth the time and money. Everything you have said so far is something that I gave you based on my own insights about myself. What have you told me that I don't already know?
> >
> > **Dr. X** *(with defensiveness in his tone)*: You act like you know how to do this better than I do.
> >
> > **Mr. W:** All I'm saying is that I have a busy life, and for me to spend time with you, I need to see results. I need to learn something I don't already know.
> >
> > **Dr. X** *(growing more irritated)*: You do not have to do this. I have lots of patients, and I don't need to have you in my practice. I'm only interested in seeing people who want to be here. I think you have to keep cutting me down again and again to make yourself feel superior to me.
> >
> > **Mr. W:** I thought the idea was that I come here and say what's on my mind. I try to do that, but then you get all defensive and act like you can't handle it!
> >
> > **Dr. X:** I can handle whatever you say, but I don't think you like to hear the feedback that I am trying to give you to help you understand yourself.
>
> Two days after this exchange occurred in therapy, Dr. X received a text message from Mr. Y: "I have decided not to return. I think you have a problem with me and can't handle me. Insulting your patient isn't what therapy is supposed to be about. Goodbye."

Luchner (2013) noted that contemptuous grandiose patients can get under the skin of the therapist with their insulting and condescending comments to the point where therapists actually unconsciously push patients toward termination through inappropriate forms of intervention. Therapists may see this pattern gestating when they start to feel a sense of dread knowing that the patient is in the waiting room or when they experience relief when the patient cancels a session.

STRENGTHENING THE SELF

Kohut (1971, 1977, 1984) wrote more optimistically about the termination of narcissistic patients. His self-psychological approach, as described in previous chapters, does not attempt to resolve intrapsychic conflict deriving from oedipal configurations. Rather, Kohut defined the overall task of the analyst as strengthening the self of the patient by finding compensatory structures to deal with long-standing self-defects (Kohut 1977). The newly strengthened self helps the patient feel more alive, more real, and more capable of feeling joy rather than emptiness and depression.

Kohut did not see the goal of psychoanalytic treatment as turning self-love into the love of others (Kohut 1984). Termination from a self psychology point of view is based on the assessment of three major constituents of the self: the realm of ambitions, the realm of ideals, and the intermediate area of talents and skills (Kohut 1984). These three domains correspond to the three selfobject transferences described in Chapter 5: the mirror transference, the idealizing transference, and the twinship transference. These three spheres are the major focus of a self psychological analysis as described by Kohut. However, progress in these three spheres may be difficult to discern because of the subjectivity inherent in assessing improvement in each area. At the end of his career, Kohut stressed that we never outgrow our need for selfobject responses, and the major change in a successfully analyzed narcissistic patient is a progression from the need for archaic selfobjects to the use of more mature selfobjects (Kohut 1984).

Being idealized may be a pleasant experience for some clinicians, and they may look forward to sessions with a narcissistic patient who will tell them how wonderful they are, especially in the context of other patients who are critical of the therapist. Patients with vulnerable forms of narcissism often are agreeable and pleasing with their therapists to avoid forms of narcissistic injury that may be inflicted by the therapist's interventions. These patients may have spent their lives trying to tune into others to figure out what they need to do to remain connected, and they may well sense that their therapist or analyst is needy of idealization (Luchner 2013). The clinician and the patient may collude in the idealization such that termination is postponed indefinitely. Therapists may even encourage further work if the patient feels that the gains have been sufficient to terminate. Psychoanalytically oriented treatments are designed to be noncoercive collaborations directed toward understanding unconscious phenomena and overcoming the various self-deceptions that have arisen in the course of development. Clinicians who engage in these treatments must be prepared to accept less than optimal outcomes (according to their own idealized criteria) if the patient feels satisfied and wishes to move on in life (Gabbard 2009).

ASSESSING READINESS FOR TERMINATION

In an assessment of whether the patient is ready to terminate, we must accept the fact that no analysis or therapy is complete. Rather, a process is set in motion that the patient will continue indefinitely (Gabbard 2009). An ideal termination does not exist. Symptoms rarely disappear completely. The patient certainly does not achieve all of the structural changes to which the treating clinician may aspire. To put it succinctly, a terminated patient is not "fully analyzed." The terminating patient is simply embarking on a life of self-analytic reflection that allows him or her to lead a richer life. Problems involving love, work, relationships, self-esteem, and vulnerability will continue.

Despite psychoanalytic mythology, transference is never destroyed or "resolved." A consistent finding in follow-up studies of terminated patients is that transference persists (Gabbard 2016). When a former patient meets with his or her former treater, transference is instantly reestablished. Neuroscience has shed some light on this phenomenon. Representations of self and others form the core of internal object relations and determine much of our thoughts, behavior, and feelings, and they are embedded in neural networks (Westen and Gabbard 2002a, 2002b). We know now that structural change in psychotherapeutic treatment does not involve the total destruction of old object relationships that contribute to transference. Neural networks cannot be destroyed. They can only be superseded by the strengthening of new models of relatedness that emerge in analysis or therapy such that the old internalized object relationships are relatively weakened.

In the assessment of readiness for termination, the analyst's observation of the patient's intrapsychic changes is continually influenced by the analyst's own subjectivity. In an era of two-person psychology, we now accept that the therapist or analyst participates in the patient's transference. Countertransference enactments are inevitable, and the "blank screen" analyst is no longer a viable construct.

Contemporary analysts and therapists know that termination involves both treater and patient in a process of disentangling themselves from a significant connection with another human being who has shaped their lives (Gabbard 2009). To some extent, both members of the dyad lose themselves as separate individuals in an analytic or therapeutic experience. Ogden (1997) notes that it is only through termination that they "retrieve" a sense of being a discrete mind. However, the mind retrieved is not quite the same as the mind that began the treatment some years ago (Gabbard 2009).

Moreover, the influence of countertransference is ubiquitous (Hirsch 2008), particularly at the time when one considers terminating. Both patients and therapists may have difficulty in letting go. We are forever vulnerable to misusing theory as a way to justify continuing a treatment and remaining attached to our patients (Hirsch 2008). Moreover, the treater's economic situation undoubtedly influences how the therapist thinks about termination. It is easy to justify one's decisions on the basis of considerations about the accomplishment of goals, the patient's capacity for love and work, and the patient's ability to continue with self-analytic process, but these well-meaning benchmarks are easily contaminated by the treating clinician's need for survival and his or her need for the creature comforts to which we all aspire. One of the greatest psychoanalytic myths of termination is that the assessment of readiness is based on a set of criteria that do not take the analyst's or therapist's self-interest into account (Gabbard 2009).

All treatments, whether psychoanalytic or psychotherapeutic, are imperfect. Terminations have to be tailored to the individual patient as well as to the dyadic nature of the process and the practical circumstances the therapist is facing (Gabbard 2009). Patients' concerns about financial issues, schedules, time constraints, and readiness to terminate must all be taken seriously rather than as mere manifestations of resistance. The clinician treating the patient can never know in advance if the patient will return for more treatment in the future. Each patient must do treatment in the way that he or she must do it (Gabbard 2000). However, when the patient decides to end treatment, it is true for both parties that the relationship matters deeply and the loss is real. Poland (2017) stressed that at the time of termination, therapists and analysts must be cautious about exaggerating the hopefulness inherent in the ending. The opportunity for a more fulfilling life and exciting future prospects does not confer immunity against future terrors. As Poland (2017) put it, "Strengths and creative potentials are to be honored but not converted into magical amulets for mutual reassurance" (p. 161).

If we apply these principles of termination to narcissistically organized patients, we must accept that the narcissism of the treating clinician is at play in ways not dissimilar from the narcissism of the patient. Narcissistic patients may systematically deny the treating clinician the gratification of a successful termination. They may need to end as they began—in a "one up" position to the treater's "one down" position. They may end with a desperate effort to preserve self-esteem by communicating to their treating clinician that they really are not that much better than when they started. Throughout the treatment, narcissistic patients may feel that it is too risky to actually depend on the therapist or analyst, and they may have to leave with a message to the clinician that they actually were not touched by the process.

Therapists who treat patients with pathological narcissism can never be completely certain if internal shifts have occurred. Patients who wish to curry favor with their treaters may mislead them. Narcissistic patients often manifest considerable skill at apparently adopting the therapist's comments and interpretations without truly changing internally. In other words, they seem to internalize the therapist's perspective without incorporating an authentic version of the therapeutic dialogue in the service of generating genuine changes in their own ways of thinking and functioning (Ronningstam 2014). Within a limited therapeutic alliance, some patients may *present* themselves as though they are collaborative, but in reality, the motives for being in treatment may be totally distinct from a serious wish to change in the areas of narcissistic functioning.

As noted earlier, some narcissistic patients cannot allow themselves to feel they are gaining anything from the process because of their intense and often unconscious envy. They must destroy whatever they receive by telling the therapist or analyst that nothing has really helped them. They are no better than when they started. A common phenomenon is that the patient maintains a view that the therapist has contributed nothing at all that is novel or different from what the patient already knew. These narcissistic resistances to a positive view of what has transpired may be hidden by an idealization of the therapist (Kernberg et al. 1989). The systematic forgetting of what the patient has learned about himself or herself in the sessions and the continual criticism of what the therapist is saying are manifestation of an envy that must spoil anything good that the patient receives.

In those cases where improvement seems to be recognized by both therapist and patient, there may be a clear indication that the direction of thinking about one's self or even *having* a self that is involved in action has undergone a transformation. On the other hand, many narcissistic patients are not able to conceptualize a self that is a source of agency in their lives. Some patients may genuinely feel less empty and more able to accept what the therapist has to offer (Kernberg et al. 1989). Gratitude becomes possible, as well as a mourning process. However, it is difficult to know a priori whether these changes are a feigned manifestation of a false self adaptation or an authentic and durable response to treatment.

> Ms. Y started analysis four times a week in her late 20s. She had worked in the motion picture industry prior to treatment and described a chaotic

lifestyle with intense highs linked to her connection with powerful char-
ismatic men followed by devastating crashes when she grew disappointed with her partners. She loved the feeling of specialness she
derived from these relationships but repeatedly found it frustrating that
the men would not behave in the way she wished. Her omnipotent control was manifested in her expectation that they would listen to her cri-
tique of how they related to her and then implement change in exactly
the way she requested. Her expectations were highly perfectionistic—
even to the point of insisting that the men should say particular words
and phrases. Even when some of them conformed to what she requested, she was still disappointed because the tone of voice or inflec-
tion they used was not what she was looking for. Men would often
throw up their hands and leave her because, as one said, "I am not going
to pretend to be someone I'm not! I can't be who you want me to be! You
can't stand the way I am and that's just too bad!"

During sessions, Ms. Y would lie on the couch and complain that no
man measured up to her expectations. She frequently said, "I'm looking
for a high-caliber man. Someone who walks into a room and commands
everyone's attention. Someone who sweeps me off my feet and makes
me feel like I'm the center of his universe." Her analyst sought to help
her see how she undermined her chances of finding a solid partner by
keeping the expectations so high that no man would qualify. He also
pointed out how her efforts to control men to make them conform to her
image of what she wanted provided no space for them to be who they
were. Ms. Y would protest and say, "But I need them to see who I am and
what I need." Her analyst clarified with her that her demand was an
asymmetrical expectation—namely, that the need went in only one direction. He asked, "Do you suppose that the man also wants you to see
who *he* is and what *he* needs?" She retorted, "I want a man who puts me
first! I'm not interested in a self-centered egomaniac!"

About 3 years into the treatment, Ms. Y became involved with Bob, a
man who appeared to care for her deeply. However, he failed the litmus
test of perfection. Her analyst cautioned her that she was at risk of losing
the best partner she had found. She started to recognize that her "selfishness" was a recurring problem in the relationship. Her jealousy of
Bob's female colleagues would lead her to explode at him for not putting
her first. Bob would plead with her, "Can't you see that the women I
work with are just colleagues?! They are not competing with you. You
have won the race. I'm not interested in them!" Her analyst interpreted
to Ms. Y that she was "deaf" to Bob's words and unable to see that he
was genuinely in love with her because he would not conform to her
narrative of what a man should be in a relationship with her. Over time,
she began to see that Bob loved her in *his* way even if it did not fulfill all
of her needs to be treated in a specific manner that would make her feel
loved and worshiped.

As the analysis progressed, Ms. Y's eyes opened to the notion that
Bob had his own struggles and that she had to make allowance for those
without rejecting him for his failure to comply with her need for omnipotent control. She recognized that she had an "all-or-none" approach to

men—that is, she had to be the center of Bob's attention or she was nothing. With the help of her analyst, she came to recognize that her demands were excessive and unrealistic. In a reflective moment, she said, "I can't feel good about myself unless he adheres to my script for him." Over time, Ms. Y came to see that Bob was there for her in different ways depending on what was going on in his life and career. She ended the analysis with a more nuanced view of her relationships and what she could expect from Bob. Her mentalizing capacity had significantly increased to the point where she was in touch with Bob's internal world. This shift heralded her readiness for termination.

Those patients who are able to use treatment to make significant changes in their narcissistic difficulties may paradoxically feel worse as they approach termination. Their attachment to dreams of glory and fame may have fended off the meaninglessness and existential uncertainty that are inherent in being human. Detaching from those dreams may initiate a mourning process in some patients who have narcissistic features. The therapist or analyst may need to facilitate this process of facing the unbearable lightness of being without the buffer of grandiose visions. The patient may come to see that those dreams were more burden than bulwark against existential despair.

THE THERAPEUTIC LIFER

Experienced clinicians who treat narcissistically organized patients know that a subgroup of these patients cannot or will not terminate. Those with serious attachment difficulties, severe early trauma, or repeated failures to connect with others may find termination such a bleak prospect that they virtually rule it out. Martin Bergmann (1997) once noted that the love experienced in the transference may be the best love relationship that life has offered the patient.

This perspective may be particularly applicable to narcissistic patients and treatments. Although the term "love relationship" may not be entirely accurate, the therapeutic relationship may certainly be the most meaningful connection that the patients have had in their adult life. They have found someone who will listen, who will empathize, who will witness their internal states and their report of external experiences, and who will make a concerted effort to try to discern the real person behind the bluster and the anxiety.

Wallerstein (1986) noted in his follow-up report to the Menninger Foundation Psychotherapy Research Project that some patients appeared to have good outcomes as long as they never had the threat of termination hang over their heads. He termed these patients *therapeutic lifers* and noted that some needed only occasional appointments every 6 months or so to maintain their improved functioning as long as they knew that their therapist or analyst would be there for them. Over a lifetime of practice, most psychotherapists and psychoanalysts who have busy practices accumulate such patients with the passage of time even though they may be reluctant to acknowledge it publicly. The mental health disciplines need to reach a point in their professional discourse where these patients are not stigmatized as "failures." For some narcissistic patients, the achievement of a positive outcome through the internalization of the therapist or analyst as classically construed may not be possible.

One group of therapeutic lifers may "terminate" in name only but continually reappear in times of crisis. In these cases of periodic returns to treatment, practical limitations of time and money may result in temporary interruptions. However, resistances to closeness and to being known may operate as well in ways that disrupt the process. The clinician needs to pave the way for the patient to return, knowing that over time there may be accumulative effects of occasional periods of treatment, leading to long-range benefits. Narcissistic patients often need to maintain the upper hand and may need to be in treatment with "one foot out the door," a positioning of themselves that assures them they will not be swallowed up or annihilated by the intimacy of the treatment process.

Narcissistic patients may be slow to change, but some research suggests that they may have positive responses to particular life events that make a lasting impact on them. Ronningstam et al. (1995) reported on changes in narcissism over a 3-year period in a follow-along study of 20 patients with NPD. Although 40% of patients remained unchanged, 60% showed significant improvement. Examination of life events suggested that three types of experiences had made a difference in their narcissistic orientation. For 9 subjects, *corrective achievements* had occurred, leading to an enhanced acceptance of a more realistic self-concept along with a diminution of exaggerated fantasies. For 4 of the patients, a *corrective relationship* had been instrumental in reducing the pathological narcissism. This observation led the investigators to conclude that some narcissistic defenses are not quite as entrenched as they appear to the clinician. Finally, in 3 of the patients, *corrective disillusionments* occurred that helped the patients gain a more realistic assessment of themselves.

The positive responses to life events are encouraging. A significant percentage of narcissistically organized patients are capable of rethinking who they are and what they are looking for. Many require more than one attempt at treatment before they can use what the clinician has to offer them. Moreover, timing may be of great importance. If they are reeling from a narcissistic wound, they be more motivated to do the difficult work of treatment and drop their defenses long enough to see what festers within them. We clinicians also need to remember that we are not the only vehicles for change and that life experience may be our ally in the long and arduous effort to help patients know themselves.

REFERENCES

Bergmann MS: Termination: the Achilles heel of psychoanalytic technique. Psychoanal Psychol 14(2):163–174, 1997

Brunell AB, Campbell WK: Narcissism and romantic relationships: understanding the paradox, in The Handbook of Narcissism and Narcissistic Personality Disorder: Theoretical Approaches, Empirical Findings, and Treatments. Edited by Campbell WK, Miller JD. New York, Wiley, 2011, pp 344–350

Freud S: Analysis terminable and interminable (1937), in The Standard Edition of the Complete Psychological Works of Sigmund Freud, Vol 23. Translated and edited by Strachey J. London, Hogarth Press, 1953, pp 209–253

Gabbard GO: On gratitude and gratification. J Am Psychoanal Assoc 48(3):697–716, 2000 11059393

Gabbard GO: "Bound in a nutshell": thoughts on complexity, reductionism, and "infinite space." Int J Psychoanal 88(Pt 3):559–574, 2007 17537692

Gabbard GO: What is a "good enough" termination? J Am Psychoanal Assoc 57(3):575–594, 2009 19620466

Gabbard GO: Boundaries and Boundary Violations in Psychoanalysis, 2nd Edition. Arlington, VA, American Psychiatric Association Publishing, 2016

Hirsch I: Coasting in the Countertransference: Conflicts of Self-Interests Between Analyst and Patient. Hillsdale, NJ, Analytic Press, 2008

Kantrowitz JL: Myths of Termination: What Patients Can Teach Psychoanalysts About Endings. London, Routledge, 2015

Kernberg OF: Borderline Conditions and Pathological Narcissism. New York, Jason Aronson, 1975

Kernberg OF: An overview of the treatment of severe narcissistic pathology. Int J Psychoanal 95(5):865–888, 2014 24902768

Kernberg OF, Selzer MA, Koenigsberg HW, et al: Psychodynamic Psychotherapy of Borderline Patients. New York, Basic Books, 1989

Kohut H: The Analysis of the Self. New York, International Universities Press, 1971

Kohut H: The Restoration of the Self. New York, International Universities Press, 1977

Kohut H: How Does Analysis Cure? Chicago, University of Chicago Press, 1984

Luchner AF: Maintaining boundaries in the treatment of pathological narcissism, in Understanding and Treating Pathological Narcissism. Edited by Ogrodniczuk JS. Washington, DC, American Psychological Association, 2013, pp 219–234

Ogden T: Reverie and Interpretation: Sensing Something Human. Northvale, NJ, Aronson, 1997

Poland W: Intimacy and Separation in Psychoanalytic Practice. Oxon, UK, Routledge, 2017

Ronningstam EF: Narcissistic personality disorder, in Gabbard's Treatment of Psychiatric Disorders, 5th Edition. Edited by Gabbard GO. Arlington, VA, American Psychiatric Publishing, 2014, pp 1073–1086

Ronningstam E, Gunderson J, Lyons M: Changes in pathological narcissism. Am J Psychiatry 152(2):253–257, 1995 7840360

Wallerstein RS: Forty-Two Lives in Treatment: A Study of Psychoanalysis and Psychotherapy. New York, Guilford, 1986

Westen D, Gabbard GO: Developments in cognitive neuroscience: I. Conflict, compromise, and connectionism. J Am Psychoanal Assoc 50(1):53–98, 2002a 12018875

Westen D, Gabbard GO: Developments in cognitive neuroscience: II. Implications for series of transference. J Am Psychoanal Assoc 50:98–134, 2002b

Index

*Page numbers printed in **boldface** type refer to tables or figures.*

Admiration, 35
Adolescents
    self-development of, 27
Age, 93
    age-appropriate displays of
        exhibitionism with empathy
        and love, 39
    aging narcissist, 135–136
    baby boomers, 22
    death and, 136
    iGen, 25
    Me Generation, 22, 23
    middle age, 64
    millennial generation, 20, 22–23
    young adults, 5, 112–113
Aggression, 38–39
Alexa, 30
Altruism
    benefits of, 11
    narcissism and, 10–12
Antisocial personality disorder, 12
    versus psychopathy, 13
Anxiety disorder, 12
Arrogance, 72
Attachment theory, 39–40
    classification of, 40
    secure patterns of, 45
Autonomy
    denial of, 35–36
    prevention of, 35–36
Avoidant personality disorder, 14

Baby boomers, 22

Benjamin, Jessica, 80–81
Bion, Wilford, 106
Borderline personality disorder (BPD),
        12, 14, 41–43
    treatment of, 98–99
        family therapy, 112
        long-term therapy in, 101
Boredom, 121–123
Bowlby, John, 39
BPD. *See* Borderline personality
        disorder
Bullying, 129–130

Casement, Patrick, 122
Charm, 38
    as a defense, 132–133
Children
    ego of, 80
    in family therapy, 113
    maltreatment of, 42
    with narcissism, 12–13
    origins of narcissism in, 44
    recollections of, 43–44
Clergy, 11, 66
Collaborative Longitudinal
        Personality Disorder Study, 42
Communication
    cyberspace and, 27
    love and intimacy with virtual
        communication, 28–30
    of NPD diagnosis to patient, 70–72
    patient-therapist, 68–69
Competitiveness, 92, 128–129

Confidentiality, 66
Confrontations, with patient, 127
Contempt, 92–93
Control, 93–94
  omnipotent, 118–121
Countertransference, 77–96
  common patterns of, 87–88
  contemporary view of, 82
  development of, 82
  with high-functioning narcissist, 86
  history with narcissistic patients,
    82–84
  influence of on treatment termi-
    nation, 146
Couples therapy, 110–113
Culture
  narcissism and, 19–31
    self-admiration as key feature
      of, 20–21
  online, 30
Cyberspace, 25–28
  communication in, 27

Death, 136
Deceptiveness, 38
Devaluation, 92–93
Disengagement, 121–123
Dishonesty, 38
DSM-IV
  diagnostic criteria for NPD, 9
DSM-5
  Alternative DSM-5 Model for
    Personality Disorders, 38
  diagnostic criteria for narcissistic
    personality disorder, 5, 7

Ego, 80
Electronic devices, 26
  narcissism and, 21
E-mail, 27
Empathy, 35, **39**
  age-appropriate displays of
    exhibitionism with, 39
  confrontation/interpretation
    balance with, 123–124

counterproductiveness of, 124
empathic admiring response of
  therapist, 89–90
for patient's struggles, 87
in treatment of NPD, 98
Entitlement, 22–25, 118–121
  management of, 67
Envy, 36, 92, 128–129
  focus on, 98
Erikson, Erik, 27
Exclusion, 121–123
Exhibitionism, 37
  age-appropriate displays of, 39

Facebook, 21–22, 26
Fairbairn, W.R.D., 79–80
Families. *See also* Parents; Spouses
  family therapy, 109–110, 112
  of young adults with NPD, 5, 112–
    113
Fonagy, Peter, 39–40
Freud, Sigmund, 82, 83

Gender, 93
  stereotyping, 14
Generational narcissism, 20–21
  characteristics of, 22–23
Google, 25–26
Group therapy, 109–110

"Helicopter parenting," 24, 43
HSNS (Hypersensitive Narcissism
  Scale), 43
Humiliation, 36, 123–124
  defenses against, 48
  vulnerability to, 37
Hypermentalizing, 46–48
Hypersensitive Narcissism Scale
  (HSNS), 43

Idealization, 36–37, 127–128
  fixed, 128
Idealizing transference, 83, 84, 90–91
  in treatment of NPD, 98
Identity, **39**

iGen, 25
Internet, 25
Intimacy, 28–30, **39**
Intrusiveness, 37

Kantrowitz, Judy, 139–140
Kernberg, Otto, 8, 109
    versus Kohut, 98
Klein, Melanie, 82–83, 92
Kohut, Heinz, 8, 83–84, 89–90, 144
    versus Kernberg, 98
    model of rupture and repair, 125

Lasch, Christopher, 19–20
Love
    age-appropriate exhibitionism
        with, 39
    capacity to, 11, 34
    virtual communication and, 28–30

Martyr
    feeling of being martyred victim, 37
    playing role of, 63
    pleasure of being, 80
MBT (Mentalization-based therapy),
    107
Me Generation, 22, 23
Menninger Foundation Psychother-
    apy Research Project, 108, 109,
    149–150
Mentalization, 46–48
    attachment and, 41
    description of, 46
    example of, 131
    explicit, 41
    hypermentalizing, 41, 46–48
    imaging studies of, 47
    implicit, 41
    patient who can't or won't
        mentalize, 130–131
    pseudomentalization, 47
    reflective function of, 41
    as theory of mind, 41
Mentalization-based therapy (MBT),
    107

Millennial generation, 20
    feeling of entitlement and, 22–23
Mirror transference, 83–84
    in treatment of NPD, 98
Models
    Alternative DSM-5 Model for
        Personality Disorders, 38
    differential susceptibility, 47
    of rupture and repair, 125
    stress-diathesis, 47
Mood disorders, 12
Mother-child dyad, 86

Narcissism
    aging narcissist, 135–136
    altruisim and, 10–12
    approach to treatment of, xii–xiii
    cultural context of, 19–31
    definition of, 10
    developmental course of, 11
    diagnosis of, xii, 15–16
    disengagement of patient with, 84
    electronic devices and, 21
    as epidemic, 23
    generational, 20–21
    "healthy," 49, 85
    heritability of, 47
    hypervigilant, 79–80, 85, 103
    key features of, 10
    malignant, 13
    narcissistic themes in cinema, 28–
        30
    nature of, 4–5
    origins in childhood, 44
    "other-deception," 86
    as overly high self-esteem, 24
    parents and, 39
    pathological versus normal, xii,
        147
    prevalence of traits of, 20
    rage and, 131–132
    research data on, xii
    sense of "lack" with, 10
    severity of features of, 12–15
    subtypes of, 43

Narcissism (continued)
  thick-skinned versus thin-skinned,
    8
  traits, 47–48
Narcissist
  capacity of to work and love, 11
  grandiose, 86, 143
  high-functioning, 84–87
Narcissistic-masochistic character,
    80–81
Narcissistic personality disorder
    (NPD). See also Transference
  DSM-IV diagnostic criteria for, 9
  DSM-5 diagnostic criteria for, 5, **7**
  families of young adults with, 5
  features of, 13
    histrionic/hysterical personality
      traits, 14
    obsessive-compulsiveness, 13
    perfectionism, 13
    self-defeating trends, 15
    workaholism, 13
  fragile type, 9–10
  grandiose-malignant type, 9
  high-functioning type, 10
  identification of patients with, 12
  lovers and spouses of individuals
    with, 6
  management of, 134
  overview, 5–6
  "pure culture" of, 13
  subtypes, 8
  with transference and
    countertransference, 84–85
  treatment, 57–75
    attachment-based, 122–123
    communication of diagnosis to
      patient, 70–72
    confidentiality, 66
    cost of, 106
    expressive-supportive
      continuum of
      interventions, 104, **105**
    first contact, 58–59
    framework, 66–68

    frequency of therapy visits, 108
    goals of, 128–129
    group psychotherapy, 109–110
    inpatient and outpatient, 113–
      114
    length of session, 67–68
    limited research on, 97–98
    modes of relating to therapist,
      68–70
    "pathologized" response by
      patient, 100–101
    patient's reasons for treatment,
      59–64, **60–61**
    patient's resistance to, 119
    planning, 106–109
    prognosis of, 140–141
    referral for, 65–66
    research, 118–119
    rupture and repair of, 124–125
    strategies, 117–138
    tailoring to the patient, 97–116
    termination of, 139–152
      examples of, 142, 143, 147–
        149
      follow-up studies, 145
      influence of countertrans-
        ference on, 146
      overview, 139–140
      premature, 142–143
      readiness for, 145–149
      strengthening the self, 143–
        144
    therapeutic alliance, 72–74
    therapeutic lifer, 149–151
      corrective achievements of,
        150
      corrective disillusionments
        of, 150
      positive responses for, 150–
        151
    when change is not the goal,
      125–127
  types of, 9–10
Narcissistic Personality Inventory
    (NPI), 22, 42

Narcissus, myth of, 6–7, 81
NPD. *See* Narcissistic personality
    disorder
NPI (Narcissistic Personality
    Inventory), 22, 42

Object relations theory, 78–80
Ogden, T.H., 80
Others
    encroachment on, 37
    loss of interest in, 38
    mistreatment by, 37
    narcissism and, 37
    seduction of, 38
Ovid, 6–7

Pain, emotional, 12, 36
Parents. *See also* Families
    attachment status of, 40–41
    of narcissistic individual, 39
Patient
    "bad-enough object," 126
    charm as a defense, 132–133
    communication with therapist,
        68–69
    confrontations with, 127
    contemptuous, 129–130
    demand for special treatment,
        118–121
    diagnosis of NPD and, 70–72
    emotional pain of, 12, 36
    hypervigilant, 14–15, 79–80, 85, 103
    omnipotent control and, 94
    "pathologized" treatment
        response, 100–101
    resistance to treatment, 119
    self-esteem, 35
    self-regulation, 35
    sense of victimization, 62–63
    suffering of, 4
    suicidality, 133–135
    therapeutic alliance and, 72–74
    who can't or won't mentalize,
        130–131
Perfectionism, 13

Personality functioning, elements of,
    39
Personality Disorder Interview–IV, 42
Personality disorders, 41–46
    Alternative DSM-5 Model for
        Personality Disorders, 38
    defenses and, 48–49
    self-defeating, 49
Personality Disorders Work Group,
    5
Positive identification, 83
Power, 93
    example of, 120–121
Praise, 44
Projection, 49
Projective identification, 82–83, 94
Pseudomentalization, 47
Pseudo self-sufficiency, 35
Psychoanalysis
    American, 82–83
    controversy of, 98
Psychopathy
    versus antisocial personality
        disorder, 13
Psychotherapy, 66
    couples therapy, 110–113
    family therapy, 109–110, 112
    group, 109–110
    randomized controlled trial for
        transference interpretation,
        100
    research support for, 125

Q-factor analysis, 9

Race, 93
Rage, 131–132
Rationalization, 48
Reality, denial of, 36
Relatedness, 33–53
    attachment disorders, 41–46
    common modes of in narcissistic
        patients, 34–38
    defenses and, 48–49
    developmental roots of, 38–41

Relatedness *(continued)*
    elements of personality
        functioning, **39**
    mentalization, 46–48
    overview, 33–34
    personality disorders, 41–46
Ronningstam, E. F., 104
Rosenfeld, Herbert, 8

"Satellite existence," 69, 89
Self
    constituents of, 144
    splitting, 48–49
    strengthening, 143–144
Self-direction, **39**
Selfies, 21
    perception of, 26
Self-importance, 59, 62
Self-love, 3–4, 7
Selfobject transferences, 83, 98, 144
Sex addiction, 63
Shame, 36, 123–124
Shedler-Westen Assessment
    Procedure-II (SWAP-II), 9
Smartphone, 26–27
Social interactions
    retreat from, 37
Social media, 21–22
    comparisons to others created by,
        25
    narcissistic behavior and, 25–26
Socioeconomic status, 93
Sophocles, 6
Spouses
    couples therapy, 109–110
    of individuals with NPD, 6, 65
Substance abuse, 12
Suicidality, 133–135
SWAP-II (Shedler-Westen Assessment
    Procedure-II), 9

Tact, 122–123
Texting, 26
TFP. *See* Transference-focused
    psychotherapy

Theory of mind, 41
Therapeutic alliance, 72–74
    building, 72–73
    collaboration with patient, 73
    description of, 72
    successful, 73–74
Therapists
    clinical challenges of, 78
        example of, 78–79
    communication with patient, 68–69
        of NPD diagnosis, 70–72
    confrontation with, 69–70
    "conned" into abdicating a
        therapeutic relationship, 91
    disengagement with patient, 87
    empathic admiring response of,
        89–90
    empathy and confrontation/
        interpretation balance, 123–
        124
    identification with vulnerability,
        91
    intolerable feelings toward patient,
        79
    modes of relating to, 68–70
    narcissistic patient distinctions
        and, 8–9
    "satellite existence," 69, 89
    "script" of, 123
    as sounding boards, 89
    therapeutic alliance, 72–74
Trait narcissism, 47–48
Transference, 77–96
    common patterns of, 87–88
    history with narcissistic patients,
        82–84
    interpretation of, 99–103
        example of, 103
        expressive-supportive
            continuum, 104, **105**
        outcomes, 99–100
        randomized control trial for, 100
        treatment planning, 106–109
    positive, 127
    selfobject, 83

Transference-focused psychotherapy
     (TFP), 98–99
   interpretative approach and NPD,
        102
Turkle, Sherry, 26, 27
Twinship transference, 83, 84
   in treatment of NPD, 98
Twin studies, of attachment classifi-
     cation, 47
Twitter, 26

Validation, 35
Victimization, 62–63

Wallerstein, R.W., 108
Winnicott, D.W., 27
Workaholics, 13
Work ethic, 22

Young adults, 5, 112–113